PERSONAL
LIFEPLAN
for
HEALTH AND FITNESS

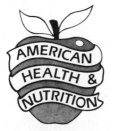

"Your total health is our concern"

We have chosen the apple as our logo, because as we have all heard since childhood, "An apple a day keeps the doctor away." It's not quite that simple, but the apple has always been associated with healthy eating and living. Of all fruits available to us, the apple has always been the hardiest and ever present, nourishing us through hard times and good.

Written by

Dennis Singsank   **David Singsank**
Health Consultants
with American Health and Nutrition

With a foreword by Leslie H. Salov, M.D.
Edited by Scott Knickelbine,
Norhern Health Communications, Manitowoc, Wisconsin

Published by
American Health and Nutrition, 7 N. Pinckney, Suite 225, Madison, WI 53703
Printed in the United States of America
Cover Design by Clayton-Davis Associates, St. Louis, MO

DEDICATION

We would like to dedicate this book to **you,** *for having the desire and willingness to seek a longer life of health, happiness and love.*

Acknowledgements

We would like to thank Dr. Michael Colgan and the Colgan Institute of Nutritional Science, as well as Dr. Tom Schulte, Hans Weber and the Alexander Medical Foundation for reviewing and giving their approval of the material in this book. A special thank you to Dr. and Mrs. Leslie Salov for all their help and encouragement.

We also want to express our gratitude to all those dedicated people working in the field of health who have contributed to the knowledge we have shared in this book.

And lastly, our appreciation goes to Jane Henneberry and the typesetting and layout staff of Madison Newspapers, Inc.

Library of Congress Cataloging Publication Data
Singsank, David and Dennis
LIFEPLAN FOR HEALTH AND FITNESS   Card #83-72757

ISBN 0-914851-00-4

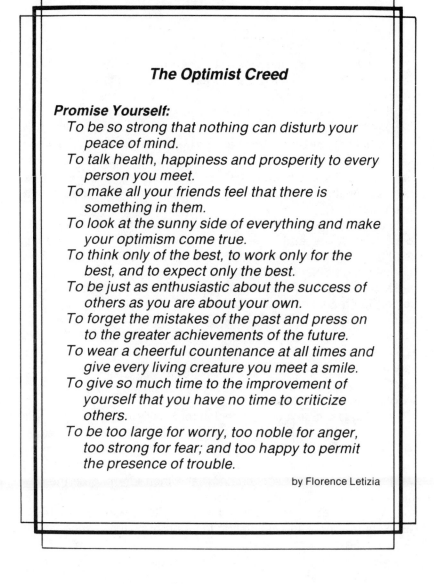

The Optimist Creed

Promise Yourself:
To be so strong that nothing can disturb your
peace of mind.
To talk health, happiness and prosperity to every
person you meet.
To make all your friends feel that there is
something in them.
To look at the sunny side of everything and make
your optimism come true.
To think only of the best, to work only for the
best, and to expect only the best.
To be just as enthusiastic about the success of
others as you are about your own.
To forget the mistakes of the past and press on
to the greater achievements of the future.
To wear a cheerful countenance at all times and
give every living creature you meet a smile.
To give so much time to the improvement of
yourself that you have no time to criticize
others.
To be too large for worry, too noble for anger,
too strong for fear; and too happy to permit
the presence of trouble.

by Florence Letizia

Because you will want to use this valuable book for reference, we have
provided this space for your personal information.

_____   _____

Name   City and State

_____   _____

Address   Phone Number

ABOUT THE AUTHORS

David and Dennis Singsank have been working in the preventive health field for the past eight years as health consultants and health educators.

After attending college at the University of Iowa, they founded WHOLEARTH NATURAL FOODS in Iowa City, Iowa which they owned until their present positions as health consultants with American Health and Nutrition, a health organization offering services and information designed to help people learn more about improving their health and lifestyle through the preventive concept of self-health care.

Over the years David and Dennis have worked with many doctors, nutritionists and other health professionals in developing healthful programs of diet, nutrition, weight control, exercise, stress reduction and other lifestyle changes for their clients. With their experience and extensive research on health and lifestyle, they have helped to create several computer-analyzed health promotion programs for AMERICAN HEALTH AND NUTRITION.

David and Dennis have written LIFEPLAN FOR HEALTH AND FITNESS to help as many people as possible learn what is necessary to enjoy optimum health and happiness.

A note from the authors:

"We suggest that you use Lifeplan for Health and Fitness as your guideline to a new, healthier, more enjoyable life. We also encourage you to incorporate any of your own good ideas into what we have presented. To gain the most benefit from this book, you may want to reread certain sections now and then to reinforce the new lifestyle changes and other healthy ways of living most important to you. You can continue using LIFEPLAN FOR HEALTH AND FITNESS for reference in helping you to incorporate these suggestions into your life."

INTRODUCTORY FOREWORD

It is with great pride that I reviewed your book **"Lifeplan For Health and Fitness"**. It is an outstanding accomplishment which fills a very critical need in the renaissance and revolution that is happening in the health field.

As a physician, practicing preventive medicine and holistic health for the past 35 years, I am besieged with manuscripts and literature from all sources, e.g., writers, centers, authors, medical, non-medical, and the associated healing professions . . . all purporting to be "the last word in restoring health."

It is sometimes difficult to wade through the overwhelming and sometimes confusing and erroneous information contained in the books I review, much of which are filled with faddist notions, impossible diets and contradictions . . . but, I am proud to write this foreword to a book which I believe is sensational.

Lifeplan for Health and Fitness is a must for those embarking on a self-help program for achieving good health and maintaining it. It is written clearly and understandably. It is medically and scientifically sound, authoritative and thoroughly researched. You have sifted through the monumental data that is saturating the health field and have seen the need for people to help themselves in matters of health. You have presented your material interestingly, simply, and in a manner which encourages and inspires one to embark on a health-achievement program.

Lifeplan for Health and Fitness will even appeal to those members of the medical community who are interested in nutritional and holistic approaches to health and disease.

As a result of your presenting me with your manuscript which has so impressed me, as well as many other physicians with whom I have shared this excellent book, I have accepted your invitation to be the medical director and educational advisor of American Health & Nutrition.

Leslie H. Salov, M.D., O.D., Ph.D.

Dr. Leslie Salov is an internationally acclaimed health educator and lecturer and is currently the director of THE VISION AND HEALTH CENTER of Whitewater, Wisconsin.

Table of Contents

GIVE YOURSELF GOOD HEALTH

Health is our most valuable asset. Other goals may seem more exciting — money, prestige, romance — but without a well-functioning body and a sound, alert mind, we can enjoy none of these things. All of us **want** good health, of course, but many of us simply don't know what to do to feel as good as we could. Yet good health is not a matter of luck or chance. It **is** obtainable, if you strive for it.

In this book you will find a direct, effective and simplified lifelong program (LIFEPLAN) explaining how you can approach total health, keep it and improve it. LIFEPLAN FOR HEALTH AND FITNESS provides guidelines to help you prevent or overcome most health problems. It will help you attain **optimum** health and fitness. Health and Fitness involve not only being **physically** in shape, but also mentally and emotionally healthy as well — total fitness of body and mind.

Every good health program will seek to establish a harmonious environment for living and working, and will include good nutrition, a balanced exercise regimen and a reduction in undue stress. Your health and fitness levels are directly related to what you eat and drink, the amount of exercise you get, the air you breathe and the everyday mental and physical stresses you experience. This sounds so simple. But often we forget how much control we have over factors that control our health. Some people get the feeling that it is useless to try to remain totally healthy and fit, but we can all maintain our health at the highest levels possible if we learn how. We can then use that knowledge in our daily lives. It is not as hard as you might think.

It is important that you do not give up trying to attain good health. Always be positive. Put yourself in command of your will power and outside influences. Enjoy your life to the fullest! All it takes is effort, patience and desire. Feeling good and looking good depend in large part on good nutrition, exercise, and attitude. "Feeling good" helps our mental attitude so much that it enables us to enjoy changing from poor nutritional and lifestyle habits to a healthier way of living so that we may **avoid** the feelings of unhealthiness.

We cannot make you healthy, only you can do that. This book can help you by giving you the knowledge you need. **You** must accept that the way to health depends on making use of the knowledge that is available to you. Gaining knowledge and educating ·

yourself are very important for true health. What you learn here you can teach others. It will give you a good feeling to know you are helping.

LEARN HOW HEALTHY YOU ARE NOW!

You can have an evaluation of your nutritional health, diet, and your entire lifestyle completed through computer-analyzed health evaluations developed by American Health and Nutrition. These thorough evaluations are called the Personal Health and Nutrient Assessment™ and the Comprehensive Life Extension Profile©. Both evaluations will help you to see a better picture of your own personal health and can act as guides when you change those eating or living habits that could use improvement. You can find further information in a later chapter.

Optimum Health And Fitness Are Lifelong Goals

When you start to change to good health habits, do not expect instant cures for problems that stemmed from years of **poor** health habits. Many people do notice changes and begin to feel better almost immediately, but this does not mean they are totally free of the problems which caused symptoms of poor health. Most often symptoms disappear first, before underlying problems are entirely solved.

Attaining perfect health is a continuous and enjoyable lifelong process, and the longer you work at it the healthier and happier you will become.

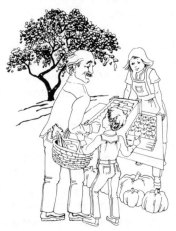

WHAT DO WE MEAN BY PERFECT HEALTH?

"Full Health is the state in which we feel best, work best, and have the greatest resistance to disease."
Dr. Albert Szent-Gyorgi, M.D., Ph.D.

Good health means to be happy, energetic, full of beauty, life, vitality, kindness, and filled with enthusiasm and eagerness for each new day. Good health means having a sound mind and sound body, smooth skin, a pleasant breath, an active yet peaceful mind, a body that enjoys work and exercise, and a mind and body that act together in a loving, true, pleasurable way.

Good health is the basis for everything we deem beautiful and worthy in life. Beauty, whether in birds or flowers, men or women, is the reflection of health and wellness.

You have the essence of health when you feel so good that you transmit waves of good cheer and happiness to others. What greater gift in life is there than being happy and extending that happiness to others?

Good health means to be relatively free of aches and pains, illness, disease, feelings of laziness, depression, stress, and other signs and symptoms of ill-health.

We must appreciate our health while we have it, not after we've lost it. We may not be able to achieve true perfect health, but we can all continually come closer and closer to that condition. The possibility of gaining near perfect health is very real. With a little inspiration, motivation, and know-how, you can easily begin to undertake a lifelong program of wellness.

"There is a lot more to being alive than not dying."

ILLNESS IS NOT NORMAL

Vigorous, robust health is the **normal** state of existence for the human race. That's **all** of us. Perfect health, exuberant well-being, vitality, energy and good-natured living should be an everyday experience for everyone. These are necessary for the realization of the highest human ideals. Anyone who does not have all of these things **now**, can continually come closer and closer to them.

Nature has provided wisely for our welfare and happiness. It remains for **us** to follow the guidelines Nature has set forth. Ailments, sickness, disease, aches and pains are not normal. Happiness and joy **are** normal. We are not put on earth to suffer. For a happy, joyous life we need only follow the practices of good health for our bodies and minds.

If you are not enjoying this wonderful, natural life, if you suffer from colds, viruses, fevers, constipation, indigestion, arthritis, skin afflictions or any other ailments, then you are not living in harmony with nature's principles.

If it were possible to measure accurately the health-impairing impact of polluted air, devitalized and non-nutritious foods, imprudent eating habits, unhealthful drinks, too little or improper exercise, overwork, destructive emotions, and poisons or toxins of various kinds, we would be appalled at the amount of abuse to which we daily subject ourselves.

Most disease is the result of external causes. Sickness and disease are not normal, although disease symptoms can be **remedial** steps to restore your body to healthfulness from abnormal conditions.

Sickness is an intense bodily purification process. Your body strives for purity. It is always trying to expel toxins and in the process continually works toward healing itself. Vomiting, diarrhea, fever, inflammation, coughing, sneezing, etc. are all processes that your body uses to rid itself of toxins. There is much we can do to help the body remove toxins. Getting enough vigorous exercise is one; drinking plenty of pure water is another.

The more we can do to avoid and eliminate the many toxins we take in each day, or that are formed as by-products from chemical processes in our body, the healthier we will stay.

BODY SIGNS

To help prevent sickness you must be aware of what your body is telling you at all times — how you look, how you feel. Pay attention to your body's signs and signals.

The word **nutrient** generally refers to protein, carbohydrates, fat, fiber, vitamins, minerals and enzymes. By reading your body signs, which often indicate possible nutrient deficiencies, you may be able to prevent illness before it occurs.

By 'body signs', we mean a combination of all the unhealthy

signs, symptoms, feelings or other sensations that most of us, including our doctors, often overlook. The body is trying to tell you something about your health through these symptoms. You may not feel "sick", but you know you could be feeling better, more energetic and more enthusiastic. This condition is called borderline **health.**

Frequently, these vague feelings of unease are linked to nutrient deficiencies. Researchers have learned about changes that take place in the body when a nutrient becomes deficient.

Some of these possible symptoms are digestive disturbances, leg cramps, canker sores, eye discomfort in bright light, scaly skin and hundreds of others.

Your body signs will tell you everyday what health problems you have and what nutrients you may need.

As you begin to understand this body language, and as you begin to learn what it means to your health, it can become the most important contribution to your preventive health program.

Your body language will tell you just as quickly when you are on the **right** track, and therefore can also let you monitor improvement.

(The Personal Health and Nutrient Assessment℗ — explained more fully later in this book — can help you become aware of any possible nutritional deficiencies you may have by cross-referencing your body's signs to specific nutrients.)

BIOCHEMICAL INDIVIDUALITY

Even if you feel you are getting enough of certain nutrients, your body symptoms or signs may indicate that you need more. There could be a number of reasons for this, including inherited genetic weaknesses or needs, poor absorption or digestion, an imbalance of nutrients which work together, or possibly any number of stress factors that cause your body to use nutrients at an increased rate.

The concept that every individual has different requirements and needs for their body and mind to function at optimum health is called **biochemical individuality.** Dr. Roger Williams, a world renowned biochemist, coined this term to denote the effect that heredity has on the nutritional needs of an individual. Paying attention to your biochemical individuality is very important. For example, some people — especially children — are unable to properly digest the protein of wheat. This is sometimes referred to as gluten intolerance or celiac disease, and may cause diarrhea, bloating and other discomforts.

Biochemical Individuality And Your Immune System

As we have just mentioned, many people have certain nutritional needs that are much higher than that of the average person. For example, those with allergies resulting from pollen or even from certain foods, usually have a much higher than average physical requirement for the B vitamins, particularly pantothenic acid. This vitamin helps to build the immune system by strengthening the adrenal glands.

Most people with allergies find they can minimize allergic reactions and symptoms by strengthening their **entire** immune system and keeping their bodies as free of toxins as possible. Your immune system can be strengthened by paying close attention to eating only healthful foods, getting plenty of exercise, drinking adequate amounts of clean water, avoiding toxins, being free of stress and its effects, and by being sure to get a sufficient amount of nutrients everyday, particularly of Vitamins A, C, and all of the B vitamins.

Many food allergies can be minimized through the proper digestion of those foods, particularly the protein in certain foods. Digestive enzyme supplements can often help to break down the proteins in these foods more thoroughly to prevent allergic reactions in your blood stream. Chewing your food very thoroughly to an almost liquid state will also be helpful. You can read more on this in the section titled "Digestion and Food Combining".

By eating some raw vegetables (including sprouts) with each meal, you'll also help your digestion by getting 'live' enzymes into your body to help with digestion and other bodily functions.

Most of us probably have **some** sort of special nutritional requirements because of our biochemical individuality.

YOUR MIND AND INTELLECT AFFECT YOUR HEALTH

Our mind and our body are all part of one unified system. When we speak of the body, we must not forget that the brain is a physical part of it. Mental activity has just as much of a physical basis as muscular action has.

Thought is one of the products of mental activity. Our thoughts affect our physical condition; our physical condition affects our thoughts. We need to care for our mind just as we do our body. We can do this partly with good nutrition and partly with pleasant thoughts arising from happiness, beauty, and pleasurable surroundings in our daily lives.

When you have self discipline and will power, you can break old habits or customs that may not be beneficial to your health, and by using your intelligence, you can then seek out those principles of health that **will** be beneficial.

STRESS AND HOW TO AVOID ITS EFFECTS

What is stress? Stress is your body's physical, mental and chemical reaction to circumstances that frighten, excite, confuse, anger or irritate you. The circumstances we refer to are those that cause emotional stress. Emotional stress in turn causes physical stress.

Stress can also be a result of physical causes such as injuries, viruses, extreme temperature change, overwork or over-exercise, toxic chemicals or certain foods. Regardless of whether the source of stress is physical or psychological, the body responds physically in much the same way.

How Your Body Reacts to Stress

Stressful situations sound your body's alarm system. Messages from part of your nervous system reach the brain, which then stimulates your glands to send hormones into the bloodstream.

These chemical reactions in your body's glands and organs (including your brain) begin to deplete your body of nutrients. Your body is trying to use these nutrients as a defense, but as they become depleted, your nerve energy is lost, your hormonal output is slowed, your immune system in weakened, headaches occur and physiological efficiency of digestion and elimination is diminished. Your body doesn't get as much nourishment and a general state of toxemia can develop. All of this, from **stress**.

"Regardless of the source of stress," states Dr. Hans Selye, "your body has a three-stage reaction to it." This prominent stress researcher has explored each stage in depth:

STAGE 1—ALARM
STAGE 2—RESISTANCE
STAGE 3—EXHAUSTION

In the **alarm** stage, your body recognizes the stress. The release of hormones from your glands will cause an increase in heartbeat and respiration, dilated pupils and slowed digestion.

In the **resistance** stage, your body repairs any damage caused from the stress. If however, the stress does not go away, the body cannot repair the damage and must remain alert.

This plunges you into the third stage—**exhaustion**. If this state continues long enough, you may develop one of the "diseases of stress," such as migraine headaches, heart irregularity or even mental illness. Continued exposure to stress during the exhaustion stage causes the body to run out of energy, and may even stop bodily functions.

How to Prevent and Overcome Stress

Since you cannot live a life completely free from stress or even distress, it is important that you develop some ways of dealing with stress. Properly handled, stress need not be a problem. But unhealthy responses to stress, such as becoming upset or angered, driving too fast, drinking too much and overeating can be damaging —or even deadly.

Although the suggestions we will make can be very beneficial, **removing** the stress will help them be more effective. Learn to avoid needless agitation when you encounter a stress situation. There is nothing you can do to change something that has already happened. Thus it is useless to get upset about it. Learn positive, constructive responses to stress situations. What has worked in the **past** to make a bad situation better and to prevent it from happening again? Think about ways you can react to the next stressful situation. Always keep a totally positive mental attitude toward **everything** in every **second** of your life.

To help you eliminate some of the stress in your life, there are several things you can do, depending on the reasons for the stress. If your stress comes from being hurried, rushed, overworked, behind in your work, etc. you must first realize that you are trying to do more than you can handle. You'll have to give some thought to lowering your sights a little and regaining your balance. Some things you can do are:

1. **Get better organized**-Know what you have to do, when you have to do it, and where the materials are to help you get things done.

2. **Establish priorities**-Make a list each day of what you must do and in order of most importance. Concentrate on one job at a time. You can't operate in high gear all the time. Remember that tomorrow is another day.

3. **"Stick to what you can chew"**-Recognize your limitations. Don't take on more work than you can handle. Other people will understand. Better to be successful at what you can finish.

4. **Be positive**-Realize that you are not perfect. Everyone has faults. If you fail, don't dwell on failure. Deliberately recall past suc-

cesses. Do not get annoyed at yourself or others when a mistake is made.

5. **Get help when necessary**-If you have any kind of problems or when you need a hand in getting work done, don't be afraid to talk to someone, or to ask for help. Confide in a friend. Each of us needs people to turn to when worries and tensions mount.

- "Talk it over." It's a healthy way of relieving tension and often helps in finding solutions.
- Remain socially active. Many people turn inward when they're feeling anxious. Social outings help keep problems in perspective and enhance self-esteem.

If stress is constant without appropriate release, the defense system becomes exhausted and you do too. A body cannot be under constant stress. Such a situation leads to rapid heart beat, backaches, headaches, ulcers, rashes, colds, allergies, asthma, colitis, arthritis, heart disease and other illness.

In fact, the American Medical Association reports that nearly 80% of the diseases that we suffer from are either stress related or stress antagonized. Also, people under high levels of stress and emotional distraction are more prone to injure themselves accidentally.

Before disease develops from stress, our bodies give us due warning with a number of common symptoms which warn us that the body is out of balance and is building up inner tension. **Stress symptoms include: irritability, tense muscles, sore neck, shoulders and back, headache, insomnia, fatigue (*not* from extreme physical exertion), boredom, depression, listlessness, dullness & lack of interest, drinking too much or developing a dependency on drugs, eating too much or too little, diarrhea, cramps, gas, constipation, unfounded fears, worrying about things you can or can't control, even worrying about the symptoms.**

Symptoms tell us we have pushed ourselves beyond a level of healthy functioning. Unfortunately when most of us experience a symptom we are apt to see it as something to worry about instead of as something we need to change.

Paying attention to yourself is the way to recognize your symptoms. Paying attention to one area of your life will draw you to pay attention to others. There are three major areas, that given proper attention, might well prevent or eliminate stress-related problems. These are healthy diet, exercise and attitude.

Probably the very best method of coping with stress is to practice a healthy life style. A wellness life style is a positive approach to living. It involves the regular practice of activities that are likely to enhance health. A wellness life style doesn't guarantee good health, but it puts the odds in your favor. It also gives you a sense of being in control. And that's important these days. We live in a time of rapid changes causing many of us to feel a loss of control over our lives. Practicing a healthy life style can help combat this feeling.

The goal of a wellness life style is to create a balance in *all* areas of life...because that's how we function best. No one can maintain a well-balanced life all the time, but the idea is to do your best, each day.

Because each of us is unique, we need to develop our own approaches to wellness.

Ways to Help Handle Stress

There are many things everyone can do to help prevent stress. Some of them, such as developing a totally positive mental attitude, have already been discussed. Other things you can do are:

(1) **Look for causes**. Who or what is at the bottom of the stress? Dealing directly with the person or issue may be the best approach.

(2) **Examine your relationships**. What can you do to put more warmth, more communication and more mutual support into them?

(3) **Evaluate**. Not every argument is worth trying to win. Defend values that are important. But learn to ignore lesser issues.

(4) **Learn to take time to relax**. At various times of the day, take a few minutes to yourself, preferably away from everything else. Sit or lie quietly, allowing your body to recharge itself fully. Especially do this when you begin to feel too much stress. Even going for a walk is relaxing. You'll have more energy and peace of mind when you return. Adding relaxation to daily life, whether for twenty minutes or five minutes, strengthens our bodies' natural resources for coping with stress.

(5) **Develop a hobby** or find a relaxing book to take to work with you or to read at home.

(6) **Create a quiet place**. Take time to meditate, to pray if you choose. Recent studies of meditation techniques and yoga show that we can train ourselves to relax.

(7) **Do something for others**. 'Reaching out' can occasionally take the focus off yourself and reduce the stress caused by brooding.

(8) **Loosen up your body** through stretching exercises several times throughout the day.

(9) **Vary your tasks or environment**, at least for short times during the day.

(10) **Use** a foot, back, or body massage tool to relax your muscles **and nerves**, or you can have someone else massage you.

(11) **Be sure to get plenty of exercise** each day. It will refresh you

after heavy emotional strain.

(12) **Get plenty of nutrition**, especially of Vitamin A, Vitamin C, B Vitamins, Calcium, Magnesium and Vitamin D. All of these are necessary for a healthy, relaxed nervous system.

(13) **Listen to soft, quiet music** at home or at work. There are cassettes and albums that are specially produced to provide relaxing music.

(14) **Having a warm cup of herbal tea** is another way to help you relax. Avoid coffee as much as possible. The caffeine can only worsen the situation.

(15) **Slow deep breathing** is also very beneficial in helping to relieve stress.

Nutrition and Stress

One way to avoid unnecessary stress is to stop eating stress-producing foods. Eating a poor diet makes us more susceptible to the effects of stress and the consequent illnesses. When planning your food intake, a good rule of thumb is to stay as close to nature as possible in your choices. Fats, refined carbohydrates, caffeine and salt are the four major foods that can cause stress to your body. Body metabolism and other bodily functions can be severely disrupted by too much of any of these foods.

Excess stress can also result in constipation. During the stress response, the intestinal functions virtually come to a standstill. Intestinal movement is reduced and almost halted. The water content of the colon is reabsorbed by the body leaving very hard and dry matter. Once this condition occurs bowel movements can be painful and difficult because of constipation.

Adding to this problem, eating refined, low-fiber foods that do not retain water within the system can cause constipation also. Constipation itself stimulates the stress response. In other words, foods which cause stress in the body cause constipation which in turn causes more stress.

When we eat stress-producing foods we reduce our body's ability to respond appropriately to the stresses we **cannot** control.

Obtain the bulk of your daily calories from complex carbohydrates. Restrict dietary fats and oils, including reducing the consumption of whole milk and other fatty dairy and meat products. Eliminate all other sources of caffeine; eliminate table sugar and other refined carbohydrates like white flour and keep concentrated carbohydrates (dried fruits and honey) to a minimum; eliminate table salt (kelp powder is a good substitute and herb seasonings help too).

Prevent Family Stress

If your stress results from caring for your children and causes you to be emotionally drained some days, there are things you too can do to help yourself minimize stress.

Probably the most important thing you can do is to have good communication with your children. Teach them about life, about their role in it, and how you expect them to help both you and your family to be happy. Children are more interested in these things than most people think. Teach them how to have self-responsibility and to take care of themselves, how to occupy themselves when you are busy with other things, and to act as peacefully as possible when they are not outside playing or in a separate part of the house. They must be taught to share and to be kind to everyone. Help develop respect between you and your children. Parents must set an example by respecting each other. The attitudes, the happiness and the love both parents show toward each other and everything they do will influence their children in the same way. Remain calm yourself at all times; don't allow violent or horror type TV shows to be watched. Whatever you do to create a peaceful environment will help you enjoy each day the way you should.

Be sure your children are eating nutritious foods (overactivity often is a result of poor nutrition). Encourage your children to involve themselves as much as possible with their education and school work, in hobbies, in organizations, or with helping around the house.

"Laughter is the shock absorber that softens and minimizes the bumps in life."

WE CAN ALL HAVE REAL HAPPINESS

Coping with stress, like other aspects of wellness, requires a sense of being in control of our lives. Each of us must realize that it is our own responsibility to do what we can to be happy.

Earl Nightingale makes this observation:

"In an excellent little book, *How to Be Your Own Best Friend,* by Mildred Newman and Bernard Berkowitz (Random House, 1971), the question is asked, People say they want to be happy; yet real happiness seems like the impossible dream. Everyone reaches for it so desperately, but for many of us it never seems to come any closer. What are we doing? Why are so many people dissatisfied in so many ways? Is it the times we live in? Do we expect too much? Do we want the wrong things? The authors, both psychoanalysts, reply, 'Too many people have just not mastered the art of being happy. They think there is something that will make them happy if they can just get hold of it. They expect happiness to happen to them. They don't see it's something they have to do. They have patience to learn to operate a car but they won't be bothered learning how to operate themselves.'

The first thing to realize in speaking of happiness is that we've probably been looking in the wrong place. The source of happiness is not outside us; it is within. Most of haven't begun to tap our own potential; we're operating way below capacity. And we'll continue to as long as we are looking for someone to give us the key to the kingdom. We must realize that the kingdom is in us, we already have the key. It's as if we're waiting for permission to start living fully. But the only person who can give us that permission is ourselves. We are accountable only to ourselves for what happens to us in our lives. We must realize that we have a choice; we are responsible for our own good time.''

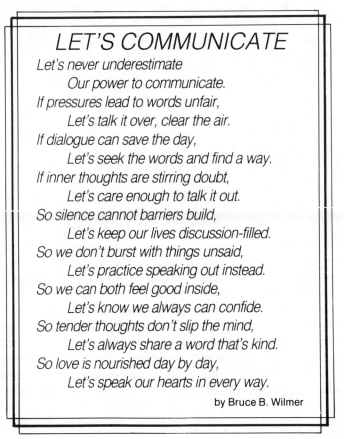

LET'S COMMUNICATE

Let's never underestimate
    Our power to communicate.
If pressures lead to words unfair,
    Let's talk it over, clear the air.
If dialogue can save the day,
    Let's seek the words and find a way.
If inner thoughts are stirring doubt,
    Let's care enough to talk it out.
So silence cannot barriers build,
    Let's keep our lives discussion-filled.
So we don't burst with things unsaid,
    Let's practice speaking out instead.
So we can both feel good inside,
    Let's know we always can confide.
So tender thoughts don't slip the mind,
    Let's always share a word that's kind.
So love is nourished day by day,
    Let's speak our hearts in every way.

by Bruce B. Wilmer

HOW TO HAVE A HAPPY FAMILY

Facing the strains of a modernized, computerized, fast-food society, people today have come to expect instant gratification. In today's mobile society, more and more people are demanding instant happiness. When we fail to attain what we want when we want it, unhappiness results. How does one find happiness? If found, how does one stay happy?

There is no single formula for happiness. However, at a time when the importance of the family is constantly being questioned, here are some facts: People who are happy live longer. Emotional discontent can lead to early aging, physical disability and premature death. People who are happy are generally more social. They have closer relationships with friends, family, clients, etc. They have obtained a sense of achievement, be it on the job or in their personal lives. Married people seem to be happier than those who are unmarried, but happiness depends mainly on the individual. Don't expect others to make you happy; relationships rely on what you put into them. Families depend on the input of all of the individuals whether it be your immediate family or a family of friends.

It takes a complex network of individual attitudes, personalities, cares and concerns to form a stable, loving family relationship. The first step in building a happy family is love. The happy marriage, founded on love, is most likely to produce happy children. The family that continues to hold together throughout the growing years is the one that keeps the loving motivation that originally brought them together. Bridging the generation gap is an important part of the process. Patience and devotion also play a vital role. Keeping your family together can sometimes be a challenge. But, despite the constant ups and downs—financial woes, job worries, husband-wife differences and parent-child conflicts, a strong sense of mutual admiration, love, trust and respect will hold the family together and keep it together forever. Appreciation and consideration are other threads that hold the family together.

Part of loving comes through expressing concern over each other's sorrows and joys. Learning what makes your sister happy and praising her for something she has done well adds to her pride and sense of accomplishment. Thanking your parents for allowing you to use their car shows that you appreciate their generosity. Similarly, attending your son's baseball game shows him that you care.

Taking time out to consider others is something we often neglect to do when we get wrapped up in ourselves. If your wife has had a rough day, ask her about her anger. Ask her what went wrong. Expressing concern over her anger demonstrates your willingness to help iron out the problems. Ignoring her feelings only makes them quietly simmer until they suddenly reach a boiling point. Comforting each other brings families through times of crisis. Loving and caring for your partner at all times and in everyday activities is the best way of creating and maintaining that internal feeling that is necessary before anyone can experience real love, and even sexual fulfillment.

Communication is also essential to building a strong family. The ability to listen to others, even if you disagree, is crucial to constructive communication. Avoiding talking about things which are problems solves nothing. If you are mad, work out the reason. If you are hurt by someone in the family, let them know about it. The importance of open discussion cannot be emphasized enough. It can make or break a marriage and can help or hinder relationships between adolescents and adults. Taking time to listen to those whom you respect may prevent a crisis or patch a difference before it gets too extreme.

One of the very important aspects of communication and continued happiness between two people is the way in which one person criticizes the other. Very often we criticize another in a way that makes a person feel hurt, inferior or even angry. We must always avoid this type of criticism. Only constructive, gentle and helpful criticism is conducive to a happy relationship. Show you care.

Part of open communication involves time. The family that plays together, stays together. Families that enjoy each other's company make that extra effort to spend some time together. If you are separated from your family by physical distance, call and write often. Keeping in touch with one's family is a vital force in maintaining relationships on the outside, too. Confidence in family relationships brings security and success in other relationships as well. No family forms a perfect web. But with a lot of love and consideration, a happy family can thrive. Just remember—there's nothing like happiness and no one will ever care about you as much as your family.

An important point to remember in order to achieve family happiness, is nothing comes easy, not even happiness. Be patient with yourself and others. Much like good health, you can't live it only because you want it or think you deserve it, you must work at it. And also much like health, family happiness requires constant maintenance and preventive care.

Take a healthy attitude towards yourself and your family and happiness will come easier.

NATURE'S BASIC PRINCIPLES
FOR GOOD HEALTH

1. Fresh, pure air is of first importance. Oxygen works like food to nourish your body. Clean, fresh air purifies your blood and helps to build and regenerate your entire body. The deeper you breathe, the healthier you become.

Polluted air, whether indoors or outdoors, will put toxins into your blood stream and begin to damage your health. There are many things you can do to minimize the amount of toxins you breathe. When driving in polluted air you shoud turn on the air conditioner and push the recirculation button if your car has one. If you are working around chemicals, always be sure there is plenty of ventilation. Stay out of places that are filled with tobacco smoke. For your house you can purchase air filter machines or negative ion generating devices, new products that will now filter the air and produce negative ions which can neutralize toxins in the air and render them harmless.

The oxygen you breathe goes to your lungs, where it aids your lungs in purifying your blood. The most important way of getting more oxygen into your body is to exercise, exercise, exercise. The more oxygen you take in, the better the health of your cardiovascular, respiratory, and nervous systems.

2. Clean, pure water is essential to the health of every cell in your body. Breathing, digestion, elimination, glandular activities and heat dissipation in perspiration can only take place with the presence of water. Even our saliva flow can become too low with inadequate water in our body. Adequate water also helps with elimination and bowel movements by causing stools to be soft and moist instead of hard and dry.

Most of us should get five to six eight ounce glasses of water daily. It is beneficial to drink two or three glasses at room temperature upon waking. At this time much of it will go directly into your intestines and will be very beneficial in the cleansing process. It is not a good idea to drink water with food as this dilutes your digestive juices. You should not drink water at extreme temperatures. When you drink or eat foods and liquids too hot, you seriously damage cells in your mouth, throat and stomach. At cold temperatures, water can interfere with digestion and is also upsetting to the rest of your body, especially your stomach and nervous system. You will find it much easier to drink water at room temperatures anyway.

A few other facts about water:

- While the average person (128 pounds for women, 154 pounds for men) in the temperate zone, may "get along" on six pints of water daily if he or she is only moderately active, two to four times as much is needed during periods of vigorous exercise or work, particularly in hot or humid weather.
- A man at rest loses over half an ounce of water through his skin every hour.
- An average human being doing light work in a temperate climate loses nearly five pints of water a day—and must replace it.

Most people need to drink more water—not more sugar-laden soft drinks or more coffee. Most soft drinks are strictly a chemical product. When sugar is not used in their manufacture, but only a synthetic sweetener, the manufacturers of such products advertise that the drink contains less than one calorie. This indicates that it indeed has no food value. Good pure water is the best answer.

Water affects our health, prosperity and joy of living. In fact, it affects every facet of our lives. Whether or not you feel good and live to a ripe age will depend more and more on the quality of water you can get.

Much of the drinking water found in most cities today is either contaminated with bacteria or chemicals, and has so much chlorine in it to neutralize the contaminants, that the accumulation of chlorine and other chemicals in your body can become toxic.

To be sure of your water, our suggestions are to buy spring water or distilled water. At an average of 75¢ a gallon it's the cheapest health food or liquid you can find. Another alternative is to buy a water filter of maybe even a water distiller.

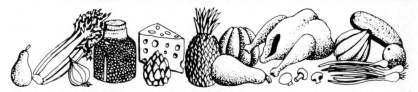

3. Pure, wholesome food free of contaminants, chemicals, additives, preservatives, and other harmful substances is of extreme importance.

Also important is the **wholeness** of the foods. Foods that have had the least processing are the healthiest—raw fruits and vegetables, whole grains, whole grain breads and cereals, brown rice, dry beans and peas, raw unroasted nuts and seeds, whole soy products, whole meats, eggs, and dairy products. However, all these foods need to be prepared properly and with care to keep them as unadulterated as possible.

The next thing to remember is to **eat a variety of the above foods** to get a full range of nutrients and adequate roughage, or fiber.

4. Sunshine is another important part of good health. Everyone knows the enormous benefits of sunshine for our mental energies. Some of these benefits are a result of physical changes our brain goes through to give us that greater sense of well being. Human beings, like plants, need adequate sunlight. Your entire body feels the additional energy and soothing, relaxing effects in its presence.

Sunshine can help to kill germs and bacteria on our skin. Sunshine is also an excellent way to obtain Vitamin D which is essential in helping your body to assimilate calcium. If you can't get much sunshine, you should at least take a multiple vitamin that includes natural Vitamin D from fish liver oil, or take Vitamin D fish liver oil capsules.

You should always avoid sunburn or heavy tanning. Too much sun will dry and age the skin, cause skin blotches, and can cause cancer. You should avoid sunning yourself between 10 a.m. and 2 p.m. for the most protection from harmful ultraviolet rays, and increase your exposure to the sun very gradually. If you do have to be out during these hours you should use an effective sunscreen lotion containing PABA, a B-vitamin. Be sure to moisturize your skin with good natural lotions after sunning to prevent drying.

5. Cleanliness, both externally and internally, must also not be overlooked. Externally, we must keep our bodies free of germs, bacteria, and chemicals. Harsh detergent soaps and cleansers, chemical mouthwashes, underarm and body deoderizing sprays, toothpastes and other chemicals we put onto or into our bodies often do more harm than good. They irritate your body's own natural cleansing process and are easily absorbed into your blood stream where they can cause many other toxic symptoms. Non-chemical body-care products or plain water are best for personal hygiene.

The main thing to remember is that proper dietary habits and hygiene minimize the need for cleansers and cover ups. Bad breath for instance, can come from poor digestion and eating habits, eating too many meat products, not rinsing your mouth after eating, not brushing your tongue daily, or from neglecting to brush and floss your teeth. Bad underarm odors are also very often a result of poor eating habits as mentioned above, and according to some health authorities, excess coffee drinking can also be a cause.

To eliminate dandruff, which is usually just dead skin flaking off, you need to brush your scalp often with a natural bristle hair brush and also wash your hair and scalp frequently with natural mild shampoo. Your scalp will stay healthier as well from the stimulation. The more you can do to stimulate and massage your scalp, the better will be the blood supply to the hair and the healthier it will look and stay.

Your skin should also be brushed and cleaned with a loofa (a vegetable fiber sponge-like pad). This stimulates your pores to remove toxins as well as removing dead skin. It stimulates and increases blood circulation, especially near the skin, and will give your skin a healthy look. It also stimulates oil producing glands, helping to mimimize dry skin. This stimulation and cleansing will refresh your complexion and make it younger and healthier. When your skin, including your face, does become dry from sun or dry winter air, you should moisturize your skin with a natural lotion.

Internal cleanliness means to have good elimination of wastes so that your intestinal environment is healthy and functions properly. Following proper dietary habits will help you considerably toward this goal.

6. Sleep, rest and relaxation are needed in ample amounts so that your entire body can be regenerated with all of the nutrients you take in each day. Your body is digesting and assimilating nutrients and removing toxins while you sleep. A seven to eight hour sleep is essential for full regeneration of your nerve energy and all other bodily functions. Short naps or periods of relaxation during the day are also helpful to maintain healthy functioning of your nerves and other bodily systems.

When you do sleep, it is important to sleep well. Some advice to follow for a deep refreshing sleep: have a soft pillow, clean sheets, a firm mattress, a healthy body, and an unclogged digestive and elimination system. A room temperature of between 65° and 70° is ideal for comfortable sleep.

People who exercise a lot require less sleep than those who exercise very little. Their blood circulation is better, thereby helping the body to replenish its energies and eliminate toxins more rapidly.

Those who need the most sleep are people who follow poor dietary and lifestyle habits. For instance, when we eat late in the evening or overeat, we need more sleep. Those who eat a lot of meat often require more sleep because of the longer digestion, assimilation and elimination of meat.

Anything that puts a burden on your digestive system at night will cause your body to be more tired and lethargic the next morning.

Excessive liquid intake in the evening fills the bladder during the night and can cause sleep disturbances. Gases, acid eruptions, and other disturbances arising from improper foods, bad food combina-

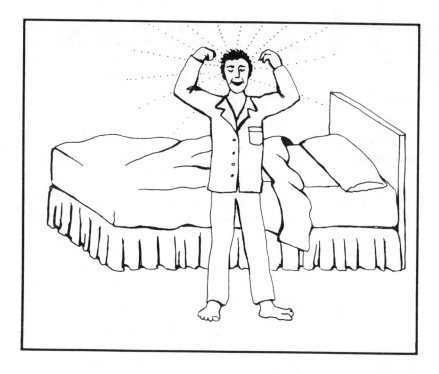

tions, overeating, eating too late, or from eating too much meat can cause your brain to be in an unsettled state during sleep. Nerve energy is lost and more sleep is needed.

For a good night's sleep you also need to avoid stimulants and drugs, including caffeine from soft drinks, coffee, non-herbal teas, and chocolate, as well as tobacco, vinegar, alcohol, aspirin, sleeping pills, salt, and stimulating condiments such as hot pepper, horseradish, raw onion, raw garlic, etc.

Lastly, perhaps the most important factor for a good sleep is to be free of worry and stress. Those who learn to control their emotions and intellect and to keep a totally positive attitude will sleep better than those who go to bed with worry and stress. If you are one of the latter, you must first try to eliminate the cause of these thoughts. If that is not possible, you must learn to put all such thoughts aside before retiring in the evening.

You must always feel confident and in control of your life. When you have that feeling, and are happy and healthy, and have followed all of the suggestions and knowledge presented here, you will wake up refreshed and full of energy, and will keep that energy all day long.

7. Comfortable temperatures, both external and internal are also important to good health. You should never let yourself get too hot or too cold, or take things into your body that are too hot or too cold. All of these things cause undue stress to your body.

8. Motivation. The happiest and healthiest individuals are those who have the ambition to achieve goals that they set and work to reach. Motivation means having dedication, purpose, direction, responsibility, and ambition to achieve your desires. Never give up hope. Remember the adage, "Where there is a will, there is a way." By developing motivation, your life will be exciting, stimulating, and never boring. We have included more on helping you develop motivation and will power in a later section.

9. Emotional Poise and **Well Being.** You have emotional poise when you feel confident, secure and socially worthwhile. These feelings are partially a result of your physical and emotional health, and partially a result of your social environment and influences, which you must always try to control or accept. Try to have a peaceful environment that makes you feel at ease. You must care about yourself, your place in the world, and be willing to keep up a healthful existence and to make a commitment to take responsibility for your health.

10. Exercise. Our bodies need more exercise than we normally get from our jobs and leisure activities. Exercise refreshes and strengthens our bodies and our minds. Lets look at the importance of exercise in greater detail.

Benefits Of Physical Activity and Exercise

1. Improved circulation
2. Lowers cholesterol
3. Tones muscles
4. Develops strength and endurance
5. Increases your agility
6. Can improve your posture
7. Stimulates internal organs
8. Helps you think more clearly
9. Reduced drowsiness and sluggishness
10. Reduces depression
11. Eases tension and stress
12. Promotes sounder sleep
13. Increases sexual motivation and improves sexual functions
14. Improved posture
15. Self esteem
16. Heightened sense of well-being
17. Helps you wake up refreshed
18. And many more

EXERCISE IS IMPORTANT!

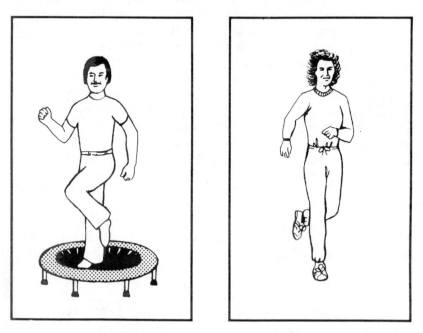

The Rewards and Benefits

Physical activity is great for the body **and** mind. The glow and radiance you see in some people (and hopefully yourself soon, as well) can be partly attributed to becoming more active and taking better care of the body. You don't have to wait a long time for the benefits and rewards of exercise and physical activity. You can add pleasure and value to your life now — almost immediately.

Exercise is as important as good nutrition to good health. Most people do not recognize the enormous and marvelous benefits of frequent exercise. If we all only knew how good it feels when we exercise, we would be a nation of healthy, happy, energetic people, from children to great-grandmothers. Regular, even daily exercise is necessary if you want to look your best, feel your best and be your best. The majority of American adults are concerned about physical fitness and are reasonably convinced that regular exercise is essential to effective performance and vibrant good health. Most of them believe exercise is "good for you" and are making some attempt to get or keep themselves in shape. Except for a dedicated minority however, their efforts are too sporadic and too limited to succeed. For example: of the 19 million adults who run or jog, one-third do so only once or twice a week, and about the same number run or jog no more than 10 minutes per outing. Here are additional findings that show the dimensions of the fitness problem in America:

- 54% of adult Americans say they don't exercise at all, and only 46% say they exercise "regularly".
- Fewer than half of all adults fully understand the kinds and amounts of exercise necessary to an effective physical fitness program.

Immediate Rewards

The immediate rewards of exercise you will be able to see in yourself:

- You will be better able to avoid or control mild depression.
- You will be able to cope with more stress, and handle it better.
- You will avoid the general feeling of fatigue that plagues so many people.
- You'll be less nervous.
- You'll have a better mental attitude toward your work, toward things in general and toward yourself; and believe it or not, you'll be able to think more clearly.
- You might have less pain from arthritis.
- You might have fewer problems with low back pain.
- You'll walk taller, stand straighter and look better.
- You'll have a more youthful appearance and increased vitality.
- You'll be slimmer and trimmer.
- You'll need less sleep.
- You'll eat less, and probably be inspired to eat better, avoiding harmful foods and eating more of the good ones.
- You'll have less loss of physical ability as you grow older. (For fully trained people, the loss of physical coordination and strength is only 12 to 15 percent from age 21 to 60.)

Remember this:

The man of 50 who says, "I can't do now what I could at 30" is often using his age as an excuse; as a crutch. If he can't do it, it's usually because he has let himself deteriorate. It is not because nature has decreed that he not be able to keep up.

The most important reward of all! Perhaps the most important of the above rewards may well be the new proud view you have of yourself — self esteem. When you feel better, when you look better, you just know you're going to like yourself a whole lot better. You're going to have more respect for yourself. You're going to be proud to look in a mirror and say, "Look at that! My stomach really is flatter!" (That comes first from tightening flabby muscles, even without losing weight.) You'll feel great about your regular physical activity and really enjoy being able to do it — a real euphoric feeling. You'll know you can do whatever you set your mind to do — it's all within you. Such a feeling of pride in yourself, a deep and justifiable self-respect might be one that you haven't had for a long time — if ever. It's one you can have again; or one you can savor for the first time.

How long does it take to get such a feeling?

It starts the first time you do something you haven't done before to improve your body. ("I did it! By George, I did it!") It grows every time you do something else. You'll love it.

Long Term Benefits

Many body functions improve at the same time through physical activity. Your heart muscle becomes stronger and should last longer. Your lungs are getting more oxygen into your blood and more toxins are being cleansed from the blood, helping your body to function better and your mind to become clearer and sharper. You will sleep better, and you will soon realize how much more energy you have when you exercise regularly.

Your muscles get toned up and become stronger, they make you feel more alive and in control and they give you a certain amount of eagerness to do things. Unused muscles wear out. Backaches, for instance, come from weak back muscles. They must be exercised or they can become depleted of calcium and other nutrients. You become weaker and lose energy. All of your seven hundred muscles need exercise, so you should do a variety of exercises and physical work each day.

Our muscles hold us together and help us to function. Some people exercise their eyes by turning them in different directions to help improve their vision. Others exercise their facial muscles to tone up their face and get rid of or prevent some of the sagging or wrinkling. That type of exercise and other types that just exercise your muscles without getting your heart and lungs pumping are called isometric. Basically, just flexing any muscle and holding it for a few seconds is isometric and will help tone your muscles.

Your bones too can be strengthened by exercise. Bones can become thin and fragile with disuse. When your body is not exercised you lose calcium from your bones.

A physically fit person is able to withstand fatigue for a longer period of time and is better able to tolerate physical and mental stress.

Even if you don't exercise to the point where your heart and lungs are working hard, you will still be doing your body lots of good, especially if you do a lot of different stretching and twisting exercises. Everyone should do gentle stretching exercises of all types every day to keep muscles toned, loose, nourished and healthy, as well as to massage the internal organs of your body, as this form of massage helps those organs, especially your intestines, to function better.

Even people who are handicapped in one way or another can find some type of exercise to get in better shape, even if it's just moving one part of their body. If you're over 60 you may not be able to add too much muscle strength, but you can add flexibility to your joints and improve the functioning of your heart, brain and other organs.

It's a fact: regular physical activity is the most effective anti-aging "serum" there is.

Lastly, regular exercise can help alleviate and prevent stress, heart problems, sickness, fatigue and the list goes on. It can even help you stop drinking, smoking, eating junk foods or whatever else you want to try to stop because you'll begin feeling so good about yourself that you'll want to do everything you can to feel even better. Many people feel they get all the exercise they need because they stand on their feet all day or have to walk around an office or hospital each day, or bowl or golf or even mow the lawn once a week. None of these activities gives your body the all-around exercise you really need, nor the overall conditioning, strengthening, flexibility you get from a good exercise workout every day (or at least every other day). After you begin giving some thought to the benefits you can get from exercise, you too will want to begin to get at least some type of regular exercise and you will enjoy it as well.

Internally some of the benefits are:

(1) A stronger, leaner heart and improved blood pumping capacity.

(2) Lower blood pressure due to better heart functioning and improved blood circulation.

(3) Lower total cholesterol in your blood and higher HDL cholesterol which has been shown to prevent heart attacks.

(4) More efficient metabolism, thus burning calories faster than normal.

(5) Better digestion and elimination.

(6) Stronger more resistant immune system.

(7) Stronger muscles and bones.

(8) More flexible joints.

(9) Stronger lungs for better breathing and blood purifying.

(10) Speed up of nerve impulses.

(11) For women — a lessening of the uncomfortable symptoms associated with menstruation.

A stronger heart and improved blood circulation will give many secondary benefits such as a better complexion, healthier skin, more radiant eyes and, most important of all, a healthier, longer life because your heart will last longer while pumping more nutrients and cleaner, more pure blood to every cell and organ in your body. Exercise increases the amount of blood the heart can pump, so it can beat at a slower rate. The lower blood pressure that results will also help your entire body to stay healthier longer as the aging process slows from less wear and tear. You will be better able to handle the stresses of modern life. The increase in nerve impulses from exercise create a healthier, stronger nervous system allowing your body's glands and organs to keep from being overworked.

By improving your metabolism (the way in which your body creates energy), you will be able to reach and maintain ideal weight while eating an adequate amount of food. The rate at which you burn calories is increased for up to three or four hours after physical activity. Digestion also becomes easier and more efficient for hours after physical activity. Even elimination will become regular and stay regular — no more constipation (assuming you are eating properly).

Stronger muscles and bones will let you enjoy any physical activity more, let you do more in the line of work or play, keep your posture better, thus giving better all around body functioning, eliminate back aches and some other aches and pains, and will help to eliminate flabby stomachs caused from weak stomach muscles. Even osteoporosis can be prevented, as bones are not allowed to demineralize.

A Few Words Of Encouragement

For those of you who just haven't been able to get it together yet to get into the routine, we want to try and give you a few words of encouragement.

First, don't think that anyone who exercises has to reach the level of perfection. Any amount of exercise in the beginning (or forever) is better than none. You don't have to be like anyone else but yourself. You may not ever look "perfect", but with adequate exercise you will definitely look better and feel better than before.

Secondly, you don't have to begin a strenuous program of exercise — at least not at first. If later on you can continue toward more vigorous exercises — great. Everyone should start out slow anyway if they haven't been exercising before.

Third, you don't have to change your whole life or become a different person than you want to be. Any changes in you or your life will come about gradually by themselves and will only be for the better anyway.

Fourth, you don't have to worry about the amount of time it will take out of your day. A lot of exercises can be done while you're watching your favorite TV program. Some of these include calisthenics, stretching, jumping on a rebounder (mini-trampoline), stationary bicycling, etc. Or you can walk faster on your way to work or school. Instead of waiting for an elevator or bus you can climb the stairs or walk. Just use your imagination about how you can incorporate exercise into your day.

Exercise can actually save you time each day in a number of ways. For instance, people who exercise don't need as much sleep since their body functions more efficiently. You'll wake up earlier and more refreshed, thus saving more time for exercise later. Plus, you will have more energy to get more things done faster. So you see, exercise certainly will not cause you to get behind in your day's activities.

Fifth, it is never too late to begin exercising — no matter what your age. Life is beautiful — if we want it to be. If there is a way to feel better while you're here, why not try and do what you can? It's not that difficult at any age to do some type of exercise.

Stronger lungs give you an increased oxygen capacity. This in turn helps your lungs to purify more blood, expelling more toxins from your body, thus providing your entire body with optimal nourishment.

We really have only touched on a small part of the beneficial physiological effects on the body from increased physical activity. And of course, the more exercise, the more benefits.

Exercise Can Be Easy and Enjoyable

There's really no reason why **EVERYONE** should not try to be in great physical shape and feel as fit as they possibly can, because it's so easy and takes so little time. With very little effort, very little time and very little trouble, you can make yourself a better person than you are now — you will feel better, look better and like yourself better. All three of those are important because you might not be completely satisfied with yourself as you are now.

Maybe you find yourself breathing hard if you walk up a flight of stairs. Sometimes you huff and puff a little getting out of a chair. Mowing the lawn or ironing the clothes or carrying in a load of groceries wears you out. You don't have much energy for anything. You're often bothered by general fatigue and mild depression. You have a feeling that you ought to do more than you are to keep yourself in better shape, but you don't know how. And you think you have to do too much.

You don't have to go "all out" with a program of running or jogging or working with weights or other devices to help yourself physically and achieve the better mental attitude that goes with it. You don't have to devote your life to fitness. We're going to tell you how you can get good results from surprisingly little effort. Furthermore, you 'll find that the things we're talking about are not only good for you, but they're fun, and they won't exhaust you or make you change the way you live in any substantial way.

Those who do try to exercise everyday already know how good they feel mentally and physically, and have experienced all the other benefits that come with it.

Determining A Program of Your Own

When it comes to exercise, your age, weight and present physical condition are all important factors in determining how much you can do. Because your program has to be tailored just for you, it must be compatible with your own needs and limitations. In the beginning, exercise should be light, increasing in difficulty as your endurance increases. Although the amount of exercise needed varies from one individual to another, the American Medical Association recommends 30 minutes daily as a minimum and states that no one can maintain or condition his or her body by working out just once a week. The workouts should be done frequently and should be vigorous enough to increase circulation and cause the individual to breathe deeply and perspire. Start with a total of 15 minutes a day — all at one time or in three 5-minute bites. Stick with that until you know you feel good about it. Then you can think about increasing the time — preferably all in one workout.

Whatever your exercise, be careful not to over do it. Beginners often exercise so vigorously that they become breathless and must cut their workouts short. As a result, they don't get enough exercise to achieve fitness. A good rule of thumb for a beginner: Never exercise so hard that you are gasping for air. When you do too much straining, your body breaks down. You become more susceptible to injury and infections. No one should exercise to the point of exhaustion. When you first begin to exercise hard, you will become exhausted sooner. You will gradually build endurance and can exercise longer, and feel better while doing it.

Regardless of your program, it's important to remember that you aren't part of an endurance competition; your pace is the one **you** set.

Keep in mind, too, that while your exercise program may not always be easy, it should always be fun. You don't have to do the things you absolutely hate. For example, some joggers consider the time they spend running, the highlight of their day. Other people can think of nothing more boring. If you're one of them, simply choose another way to fill your activity requirements.

The key to the success of any exercise plan is, of course, consistency. To get maximum benefits, you have to exercise on a regular basis. Just as start-and-stop crash dieting has little long-term value, sporadic exercise isn't much good either. And while you needn't join a gym or invest in a lot of expensive equipment, you do need to set a specific time aside each day, and refuse to let anything else interfere. Make exercise one of the high-priority items on your daily schedule. Exercising once a week yields only sore muscles; pick activities that can be done regularly. They needn't be the same ones every day; in fact, variety adds spice to an exercise schedule.

The Exercise Best For You

Many people ask if any one exercise is better than another. Again, that depends on your own needs and limitations. Still, some authorities say swimming is the best single thing you can do, because while it exercises all the muscles, body weight is buoyed up by the water.

Walking is also good because it's a fine conditioner, bringing nearly every muscle into play. And of course, it's free and can be done by people of all ages.

Jogging is another all-around muscle exerciser, but should be undertaken only after checking with your doctor. Running in place is another good exercise, especially when outside weather conditions are not good.

Some people prefer working out with a jump rope, which is simple and convenient. According to **Prevention** magazine, 10 minutes of brisk jumping or skipping rope is equivalent to 30 minutes of jogging.

All of the above are good for exercising the leg muscles, which many of us don't do frequently enough.

The new mini-rebounder trampolines on the market have many beneficial effects on your body that other forms of exercise do not offer. Most importantly, the up-and-down anti-gravity action activates your lymph system, and helps to eliminate toxins from your blood at a faster rate than normal. Begin a mini-tramp exercise program with ten minutes of jumping every day, and gradually build up to 20 minutes or more. Start and end each session with a minute or two of very slow jumping. But you don't have to just bounce up and down. You can also: jog, kick forward or out to the side, hop from side to side, do jumping jacks — or use any other special bouncing techniques that occur to you (as long as they're easy and safe). These 'mini-tramps' are fairly inexpensive and can give you a chance to get good aerobic exercise indoors. They are actually a very fun way of getting exercise. Perhaps the best thing about the rebounder is that it's an excellent way of getting aerobic conditioning in the winter and still stay warm.

Bike riding is popular and is also an excellent family activity. And don't forget about recreational sports, such as tennis, golf, racquet and handball — whatever you enjoy, within reason.

Just be sure that you take a comon sense approach to exercise, because sudden exertion can increase the heart's workload as much as five times the normal. Any exercise you can do is healthful, as long as it is a good and varied amount each day, or at least as often as is possible.

Other new health promoting products available are the anti-gravity devices. By hanging upside down, people have been relieved of backaches and other problems that are a result of constant compression of our bodies. Upside down anti-gravity action helps your skeletal system, especially the back and spine, as well as your internal organs and brain. Because the increased blood flow carries nutrients and oxygen to your brain, your thinking will become clearer too. The increased circulation to the scalp may also reduce hair loss.

Most exercise and physical activity can be done in or around your own home. Of course, alternatives can be employed. If you enroll in a keep-fit program at the Y, in the school, the recreation center, or the club, the home routine can be skipped on the meeting days. On those days when there is no class, follow the do-it-yourself program. Those fortunate enough to have the time and facilities for sports should by all means take part.

To Help You Get Started

(1) Plan your exercise schedule. Set some specific time aside each day — don't leave it to chance.

(2) Let others help you. Let your family and friends, even co-workers know you plan on getting into an exercise program. They can all give you encouragement and perhaps even join you.

(3) Reward yourself. If you stick with it, give yourself little (or big) rewards now and then to reinforce your self-discipline.

You will also find that once you accept the self-discipline of an exercise program, it will be easier for you to moderate other habits. People who start taking better care of their bodies tend to stop or cut down their smoking, and stop eating the wrong foods and choose more of the right ones. They often become more interested in taking care of themselves, read articles they wouldn't have read before and educate themselves on the advantages and the ways of building better health.

Should You See A Doctor First?

As long as you begin your exercise program slowly, you really don't have to consult your doctor first. However, if you smoke cigarettes, have high blood pressure, if you know you have joint problems, heart problems, leg pains or diabetes, or other health problems, you should first see an exercise-oriented physician and discuss what you plan on doing. Ask for adivce and assistance before starting a vigorous program.

If you can't stop smoking altogether, don't smoke less than 20 minutes before exercise. Women whose menstrual periods stop altogether may want to cut back on exercise, as hormone levels may be altered too much due to too much reduction of body fat. If you haven't exercised in a long time, be sure to start with just a few minutes a day and gradually increase that time. Also, be sure to warm up with stretching exercises before you begin. Before you do begin, it's a good idea to keep the following guidelines in mind:

(1) Decide whether you prefer group or individual activities.

(2) Select a sport or exercise activity you find enjoyable and look for a class or location in which you find a comfortable atmosphere.

(3) Select an activity that is challenging, but not overly demanding in keeping with your present physical capabilities.

(4) Be sure that you like the people you are exercising with — especially if it's a small class or a one-on-one sport.

(5) Do a little research on your own. Find out which exercises are good for your body and which are not.

(6) CONVENIENCE is the most crucial aspect of any regular physical activity. If you live and work too far from the place, you'll find it easy to skip sessions. Is the activity you've chosen one that you can participate in during all seasons?

How Hard Should You Exercise?

Give yourself a few basic tests to determine your body condition, then choose your activity accordingly. Always do warm-up and circulation exercises regardless of your fitness level.

Circulatory-respiratory fitness is measured by counting the number of heart beats (your pulse rate) per minute. Monitoring the level of effort you put into exercise or sport activity is the safest way to be sure you do not overtax your heart. This test will give you a good idea of your present physical condition and act as a gauge as you progress in your fitness program.

The **best** way to know you are exercising properly is to take your pulse before, during and after your exercise session. Most adults have heart rates of 60 to 75 beats per minute while at rest. Raising this to 120 beats per minute or more indicates adequate exercise for most people. Sustaining activity at this level for 15 minutes three times per week is known to benefit the heart. This should represent the absolute minimum routine exercise program. An optimal program would be approximately 30 to 45 minutes per day, but this much time three times per week is probably adequate. Getting 30 to 45 minutes per day is probably easier than you think. It is a matter of believing exercise is important, and then taking advantage of stairs, walking, and so on to get in the needed minutes within your routine.

As you get into shape, you will note that **(1)** your resting heart rate is lower, **(2)** it takes more exercise to raise the heart rate to 120 beats per minute, and **(3)** your heart rate returns to the resting rate more quickly following exercise. This indicates that muscles, heart and lungs are becoming more efficient and effective. If you're in normal health, your pulse will indicate immediately whether or not you are exercising within safe limits. While exercising vigorously try to bring your pulse rate to 70 to 80 percent of maximum. To find your maximum, subtract your age from 220. Therefore, your pulse during exercise should be approximately:

147 if you are 10 years old;
140 if you are 20 years old;
133 if you are 30 years old;
126 if you are 40 years old;
119 if you are 50 years old;
112 if you are 60 years old;
105 if you are 70 years old.

This is using the 70% rate. To calculate your own physical stress limits, subtract your age (say 59) from 220. The answer is 161 beats per minute (bpm), the maximum possible heart rate for a person aged 59.

Next, calculate 80 percent and 70 percent of 161. For a 59 year old person, eighty percent is 129 bpm, the upper limit of the "training effect" zone. A person of 59 should never exceed this limit when exercising unless optimally fit. Seventy percent is 113 bpm, the lower limit of the "training effect" zone.

To take your pulse, count the number of beats during a 15-second period and multiply by four.

For anyone between 30 and 55 a quick way to tell if you are "overdoing it" is this: after exercising, rest for exactly one minute. If you pulse registers over 130 bpm, reduce your pace and distance until your pulse registers closer to 100. If after resting five minutes your pulse registers over 120, this is a definite sign of over-exercising. If after resting for ten minutes your pulse registers over 100, this also confirms that you are pushing yourself too hard. These figures should be gradually reduced for persons over 55.

Once you are in condition, but not before, you should strive to keep your pulse in the "training effect" zone during exercise. For a 59 year old person this is between 113 and 129 bpm. Always stay within safe limits as you gradually increase your pace and distance until you are spending a maximum of thirty minutes at a time in the "training effect" zone. There are small, convenient, computerized monitors available to help you calculate your exercise rates.

Numerous studies have shown that by exercising to the point where "training effect" is experienced for at least thirty minutes three times or more each week, you will experience a tremendous increase in heart and lung power, in oxygen uptake, and in energy, stamina and endurance.

Categories of Exercise

There are three categories of exercise — all very beneficial and important. They are warm-up, muscle strengthening, and aerobic endurance.

WARMUP EXERCISE

Warmup exercises are necessary before and after any strenuous exercise activity. The latter is more appropriately called cool-down. The warmup exercises start the oxygenated blood flowing to your muscles. This will warm and stretch the muscles to prevent injury and will make your whole body feel more invigorated for more strenuous activities. Your heart rate, respiration (breathing) and body temperature will also increase. Cool down prevents muscles from tightening up. The best type of exercises for both warmup and cool-down are the stretching and bending exercises. They will also help to tone your muscles and add flexibility. When stretching and bending it is best to do this slowly without bouncing. Doing slow jumping jacks or some brisk walking should precede stretching to promote blood circulation and warming of the muscles. Avoid **deep** knee bends as they can damage the joints. Also to prevent knee damage, keep your knees bent when touching toes or doing sit-ups. Holding positions for ten to thirty seconds will give the most benefit. The warm-up period should be 10-15 minutes.

Following are some very good warm-up and cool down exercises that will prepare your body for your daily exercise program or favorite sport.

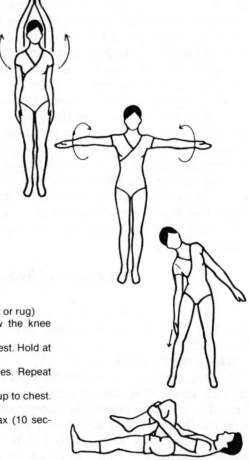

Deep Breathing
Inhale fully as you raise arms from front to overhead position. Lower arms to your sides while exhaling fully. Repeat 10 times.

Arm Circles
Extend arms to the side and rotate in tight (6") circles, reversing direction after 10 counts. Repeat twice.

Side Bends
Bend to one side with a slow, stretching motion as your arm reaches down the side of your leg-hold and relax. Alternate stretching one side and then the other. Repeat 5 times each side.

Low Back Exercise (use mat or rug)
Lying on back, grab below the knee with both
hands and bring knee to chest. Hold at least 10
seconds or until back relaxes. Repeat with other
leg. Now, bring both knees up to chest. Hold
until low back muscles relax (10 seconds).
Repeat 3 times.

Curl-Up

Lying on back, knees bent so that feet are within 12-18" of buttocks, hands clasped behind head. (Place feet under sofa for support.) "Curl up" toward knees, lifting head, shoulders, and back in that order. Note: If you cannot "curl up" with hands behind head, hold arms straight out in front of you. Repeat 5-10 times, depending upon state of fitness.

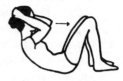

Flexed-Leg Back Stretch

Starting position: Stand erect, feet shoulder width apart, arms at side. Action: Slowly bend over, touching the ground between the feet. Keep the knees flexed. Do not look at them. Hold for 10 to 15 seconds. If at first you can't reach the ground, touch the top of your shoe line. Repeat 2 times.

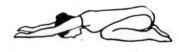

Lying-Hamstring Stretch

Lying on back, raise one leg as high as you can toward the ceiling. Repeat 5 times for each leg.

Back Stretcher (use mat or rug)

On hands and knees, slowly slide back until you are sitting on heels with palms still on floor, arms straight, head down. Come up to starting position, arching back slightly. Repeat 5 times.

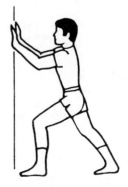

Leg Stretch

Face wall. Placing one foot in front of the other, keep back leg straight and lean forward until you feel stretched in the calf. Reverse leg. Repeat 5 times.

MUSCLE STRENGTHENING EXERCISE

The next category of exercise consists of those that strengthen your muscles. These might be pushups, weight-lifting, sit-ups, knee bends, leg lifts, etc. Doing a variety of sit-ups can help to strengthen abdominal and back muscles thereby helping to tighten a flabby stomach and relieve back pain. Strengthening the stomach muscles will help to eliminate the so-called middle-age spread. You can even get a pair of dumbells for your home or office, or even better there are now small compact hand-comforming weights available that can really help to strengthen the entire top half of your body. One such type is called "Heavy Hands". You can also get aerobic exercise from these exercises if you keep weights light enough to do a lot of repetitions.

Conditioning Exercises For Men and Women

Abdominal

Select the one for you.

Head and Shoulder Curl:
Starting Position:
Lie on back, legs straight, arms at sides
Action:
Count 1—Curl head and shoulders off floor.
           Hold this positionfor 5 counts.
Count 2—Return to starting position.
Suggested repetitions: 10-15

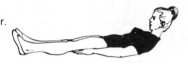

Situp, Arms Crossed:
Starting Position:
Lie on back, arms crossed on chest,
hands grasping opposite shoulders.
Action:
Count 1—Curl up to sitting position.
Count 2—Curl down to starting position.
Suggested repetitions: 10-15

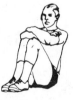

Arms and Chest

When doing these exercises, keeping the back straight is important. Start with the knee pushup and continue for several weeks until your stomach muscles are toned up enough to keep your back straight. Then try the intermediate.

Knee Pushup (beginner)
Starting Position:
Lie prone, hands outside shoulders, fingers pointing forward.
Action:
Count 1—Straighten arms, keeping back straight
Count 2—Return to starting position.
Suggested repetitions: 5-10

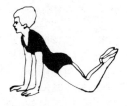

Quarter Knee Bends
Starting Position:
Stand erect, hands on hips, feet comfortably spaced.
Action:
Count 1—Bend knees to 45°, keeping heels on floor.
Count 2—Return to starting position.
Suggested repetitions: 15-20

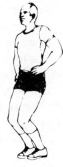

Pushup (intermediate)
Starting Position:
Lie prone, hands outside shoulders, fingers pointing forward, feet on floor.
Action:
County 1—Straighten arms, keeping back straight
Count 2—Return to starting position.
Suggested repetitions: 10-20

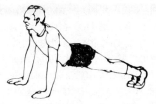

AEROBIC (ENDURANCE) EXERCISE

Aerobic means "with air". While other exercises benefit only your muscles, aerobic exercises get your cardiovascular system into shape as well. If you exercise vigorously for more than 2 to 3 minutes, your muscles need oxygen to keep generating energy. Aerobics makes your heart more efficient at getting oxygen to your muscles and your muscles more efficient at using the oxygen to produce energy.

To get the BENEFITS of aerobic exercises you must exercise continuously for 20 to 30 minutes at least three times per week. The benefits referred to are those mentioned in an earlier section — strengthening of the heart, lungs, glands, and other organs, along with beneficial effects on just about every other bodily process. Some of the best types of aerobic exercises are brisk walking, jogging, bicycle riding, a strenuous weight workout, swimming, running, aerobic fitness and dance classes, or cross country skiing.

Various exercises affect the body somewhat differently. For best effect, vary your activities. All of your muscles are important. An exercise program should be balanced just as a diet should be balanced. Some parts should be designed primarily to exercise the heart and lungs in a way that will develop endurance.

Other parts of the program should be directed toward the improvement of strength, agility, flexibility, balance and muscle tone.

Whatever the exercise, be sure to replace the fluid you lose through sweat by drinking plenty of water.

Yoga - Stretching and Flexibility Movements

For spinal flexibility, muscle stretching, breath control and mental relaxation, no exercise surpasses yoga. There is a lot more to yoga than warm-up, stretching and flexibility-type exercises or movements, but this is the part of yoga that can get your body ready for other physical activity and at the same time tone up your muscles, internal organs and add flexibility to your spine. Basic to all yoga is learning to breathe in a special, healthier way — deeply and slowly. There are many books available on this subject.

Walking

Health experts agree that walking is one of the best over-all physical activities for the body. However, the brisker the walk, the better — something more than a stroll, as though you intend to get somewhere. Stand erect and walk tall. Keep your chin up. Swing your arms vigorously and use a long, flowing stride. Walk to work, walk around the block, even around the inside of the house and up and down the stairs. Walking 45 minutes a day can help you lose or keep off up to 30 to 35 pounds a year — if you are overweight.

Brisk walking exercise is excellent to help overcome fatigue, depression, stress and anxiety. Even headaches often go away when walking. Walking is a perfect aid to digestion, elimination and circulation.

Before starting a walking program, be sure you have a pair of comfortable, cushioned, flexible shoes, and wear comfortable clothes.

The Footwear Council has a booklet that promotes plenty of tips about how to start walking for the purpose of serious exercise. You can get a copy of this well-illustrated and informative booklet by sending $1.00 to The Footwear Council, 720 Fifth Avenue, New York, NY 10019.

Jogging

It's true that jogging isn't the only sport that improves health — but it is one of the best. Why?

Jogging burns about 400 calories a half-hour — the amount in a hot-fudge sundae. You need little equipment and no special athletic ability. You can jog almost anywhere, anytime, with a friend or without. You can jog outside in the fresh air — and a few minutes of outdoor exercise can clear your mind and change a bad mood to good. However, try to avoid areas with heavy traffic or pollution.

Jogging can give you all of the benefits of other aerobic exercise. Personally, it is our favorite aerobic activity, along with rebounding, swimming and bicycling. 10 to 15 minutes of stretching and calisthenics, a few minutes of pushups, and another 10 to 20 minutes of jogging three to six times a week can make you feel as good as you want to be. What's best is what's comfortable for you. Although comfort is the most important factor, there are a few specific points about posture that can make jogging easier and more fun.

● First of all, run tall. Keep your back fairly straight and your head up. Look ahead, rather than down at your feet.

● Relax your body — neck, arms, hips and ankles. Your arms should be bent at about a 90-degree angle. Keep your hands loose. Clenching your fists can cause tension in other parts of the body as well.

● Breathe through your mouth with your mouth slightly open. Use your stomach and lower abdomen muscles, rather than the muscles of your chest.

● Make sure you land on your heels, or even flat-footed, rather than on your toes. Running on your toes can give you sore calf muscles and shin splints and it is more tiring.

Don't feel that you have to take long strides. Some of the best (and fastest) runners have what is called the shuffle stride. Shufflers seem to "skitter" across the road using short, rapid strides, little knee lift and little kickback. There is a good reason for using the shuffle. It's the stride that's easiest on your legs. To do it, begin with a walk, and gradually increase your speed (but not the length of your stride) until you are forced into a run. Keep that pace, or go faster. If you are "shuffling" correctly, your feet will seem to slide across the ground instead of lifting. A minute or two of brisk walking before and after jogging will help you limber up and stay limber. The main secret for correct form is — don't strain. Run easily and naturally. And don't worry, either. The more you jog, the easier it will become.

Cautions:

You should stop immediately when you feel any local pain. One of the most common pain-causing mistakes made by beginning joggers is thinking they have to run every day. If you're tired from yesterday's run (jog), don't beat yourself into the ground. Jog at a level that leaves you relaxed and energetic, not pooped.

Pain may also come from not being able to breathe easily. In that case, slow down. Even stop and walk. If you're so out of breath that you could not converse with a friend while running, you're going too fast.

Prevention-minded physicians recommend that we tune in and listen to our bodies for any signs that we are overdoing it. Thus a person in normal health is advised to begin with a brisk daily walk. Then gradually increase your pace and distance. When you can walk five brisk miles without fatigue, you'll probably feel ready to jog. Start by alternately jogging fifty paces and walking fifty paces. After only a few weeks, many people find they can easily jog three miles in thirty minutes.

Running

Running has been taken up by a large number of people as a preferred form of physical activity. However, this activity has also produced the largest number of injuries, especially of the knees, joints and tendons. If you are going to run, be sure to have good shoes, run on flat surfaces (preferably soft), and keep your distances reasonable. Two to 3 miles a day is sufficient. Remember, the harder you land the more wear and tear on your tendons and joints. Also, be sure to warm up with stretching exercises. If you feel pain or pressure in the chest, stop and rest. The same applies to pain in your back or legs. The key to running is to make it safe and fun.

Jumping Rope

Jumping rope is fun, convenient, and inexpensive. It saves time, strengthens the heart, improves your skill at sports, reduces nervousness, increases endurance, and helps reduce weight. And the beautiful thing about jumping is that it's easy to do, almost any time and any place.

In terms of overall fitness, most exercise physiologists agree 10 minutes of non-stop jumping is equivalent to 30 minutes of jogging, as far as all the aerobic effects are concerned.

Jumping rope is an excellent way to exercise the heart and lungs as it is a rhythmic exercise which may be started gradually and then developed into a demanding workout. Thus, its benefits are similar to other aerobic or endurance-type exercises. Physiologically, jumping rope also benefits the muscles, the digestive system and general appearance.

The motions of hopping, skipping and jumping not only increase circulation throughout the body, but also aid in peristalsis (the movement of material through the digestive system) in a natural way. Regularity need not come in a bottle or tablet; it is a natural part of our make-up, built into our miraculous bodies if we exercise them.

For free literature on guidelines to easy and effective jumping, write to: Jumping for Fitness, PO Box 636, Newton Lower Falls, MA 02162.

Swimming

Swimming is an activity that can tone and strengthen more muscles than almost any other activity and does wonders to build lung capacity. It does not help too much with the abdominal and lower back muscles however. Swimming causes no stress on the bones. If possible, try to swim in a nonchlorinated pool or one with minimal chlorine. For maximum effect, use a variety of strokes and do some 'treading water' as well.

The Joy of Bicycling

Like walking, swimming and running, bicycling on a regular basis provides many of the elements of an effective physical fitness program. It may just be the most pleasant exercise of all.

Bicycling can be done almost anywhere: on city streets that have bicycle lanes, in parks, on roads, even in shopping mall parking lots before and after hours. With geared bicycles, almost no hill is too steep, no incline too long to be conquered!

Health Clubs - For Exercise

Health clubs are a great place to take part in a variety of exercise activities all in one place. Most have aerobic dance and fitness classes, weight lifting equipment, slant boards, rebounders (mini-trampolines) and often you'll find a swimming pool and perhaps a gymnasium, sauna and whirlpool for sore muscles.

Perhaps the best aspect of exercising at a health club is the individual attention you can often get — for the asking. Another benefit is that you can exercise with other people if you wish. This can sometimes help if you need the extra motivation. There are many different types of health clubs available including YMCA's and YWCA's, so you shouldn't have any problem finding one to suit your needs.

Aerobic Exercises and Dance

This type of physical activity is very good exercise for building the aerobic capacity of your body as well as for improving flexibility. These classes are usually held in your community recreation center, YMCA or YWCA, or local health club. This form of aerobic exercise is excellent for staying in shape in almost every way and best of all, can be lots of fun. These fitness classes are almost always accompanied by music that keeps you exercising naturally with the sound. It is also a good way of meeting other people.

Weight Lifting

In order to build larger and stronger muscles in your legs, arms, back, shoulders, stomach, chest, etc. you need not necessarily lift weights, but a good program of "weight lifting" can probably build and strengthen these muscles faster than anything else you could do.

Stronger muscles can not only give you more strength and endurance, but when combined with a good stretching program can help to prevent injuries to your body from other physical activities. Most weight-trained athletes also say that lifting weights provides for a greater measure of self-confidence. Greater strength and self-assurance can make you better at whatever physical activity you engage in, and you will not tire as easily either, thus making your activity more enjoyable.

The best type of weight lifting equipment to look for in a health club is the 'progressive-resistance' type which is safer and more effective.

Ask one of the health club staff for more details on what type of workout is best for you. We suggest that if you do include weight lifting in your exercise routine that you be sure to not overdo this activity as it can put too much stress on the heart, as well as raising the blood pressure tremendously. A variety of all types of exercise is best.

More Exercises For the Elderly — or Anybody Just Starting Out

Walk briskly for two minutes around a room.

From two to 10 times, bend over slowly, bending your knees, and try to touch your fingers to the floor. Don't worry if you can't do it at first — or ever.

Rotate your head two to 10 times in each direction. Do it sitting at first, in case it makes you dizzy.

Stand with your back against a wall, your feet six inches from it. Tighten your buttocks and stomach muscles and press your hips, spine and shoulders against the wall for 15 seconds. Relax for 15 seconds.

(To count seconds, count "One thousand one; one thousand two," etc.)

Hold your arms straight out to the sides. Make large circles with both arms, five times in each direction.

Hold your hands straight out in front of you, shoulder high, then swing them back as far as possible on both sides. Do it two to five times.

Lie down on the floor. Bring each knee up as close to your chest as you can, two to five times.

Lie on your side with one arm straight up. Then lift your upper leg, keeping it straight. Do it two to five times. Roll on your other side and do the same thing with the other leg.

Lie on your back and lift your head and shoulders and your feet and legs off the floor, balancing on your buttocks. Hold for four seconds. Do it two to five times.

Other Simple Exercises Anyone Can Do

Lying in bed (perhaps to start your day), stretch your whole body, with your arms over your head and your legs extended. Hold for five seconds, then relax. Do it several times.

Do situps in bed, reaching toward your toes.

Hold the edge of the kitchen counter, a desk or the back of a chair and lift each leg behind you and stretch it slowly, raising it as high as you can. Alternate legs.

While sitting, suck in your stomach and tighten your buttocks as hard as you can. Do not hold your breath. Hold for five or six seconds. Relax and repeat.

Put your hands on the chair arms or the seat beside you and slowly lift yourself up a few inches. Hold for five seconds and let yourself down slowly.

Make a tight fist and hold it. Relax and repeat.

While sitting, grab one knee with both hands and pull it toward your chest. Alternate knees. Then do both at once.

While standing, rise up and down on your toes.

Sitting down, hold your feet out in front of you and make circles at the ankle. Rotate your feet away from you and then toward you.

(You've got joints in your arms, legs and neck. Each one ought to be moved through its full range of motion every day.)

Stand straight and swing each leg forward and then back six times.

Keeping your head straight, shrug your shoulders up to your ears, one by one and both at the same time.

Lean forward and touch your toes while standing. Keep your knees slightly bent. You can also do this one while sitting on the floor with your legs straight out in front of you.

Stomach Flattener

To help strengthen your stomach muscles even faster than with regular sit-ups, try doing sit-ups on a slant board or make your own out of a board covered with padding with an object set up under one end. By lying with your head on the low end and then doing sit-ups and leg lifts, the force of gravity can help to get rid of the extra flab in your stomach area (of course, regular aerobic exercises and attention to diet are also necessary.)

One stomach exercise that perhaps works even better to strengthen the stomach muscles is as follows:

Lying completely relaxed in the slant position, draw in your stomach as you count one. (Continue breathing naturally while doing this exercise.) Draw your stomach in and up, farther, on the count of two. On the count of three you draw it in close to your spine, which is pressed flat against the board. Try to hold this position to the count of 10. Then relax. Repeat the exercise as often as you wish. This exercise is the **stomach lift.**

Do the stomach lift for the rest of your life, and save your waistline permanently. You will be saved from sagging shoulders, flabby stomach and have a strong, permanent "muscle corset" supporting the center of all the vital processes of your body.

Master the stomach lift, and when you walk you will keep your stomach flat without effort. Take long steps when you walk, feel the good, rewarding "pull" in the muscles of your legs and buttocks, feel your shoulders go back, hold your chest high, feel your neck straighten and carry your head proudly.

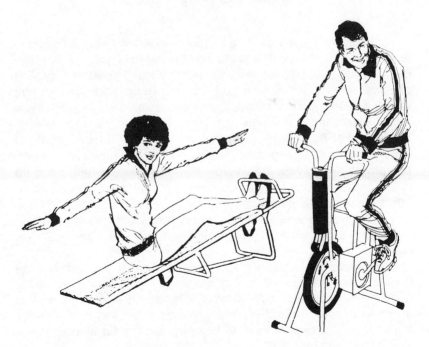

Exercise Equipment Can Help, Too

Once you get involved and perhaps want to do a little more, there is good equipment available for not much money that you can use in your home. The most popular are the rebounder, stationary bicycle, treadmill, rowing machine and dumbbells. Don't rush out and buy one until you're sure you want it and will use it. Too many people find that writing the check and assembling the machine satisfies their need for physical activity. Don't kid yourself.

Don't overdo it at first. Start slow and build.

Whenever you're doing something in the activity line at home, it's a good idea to do it with music. **Music adds rhythm and can make your exercises more enjoyable.** It can give you something to think about other than what you're doing.

Exercise and Weight Control

Probably the most important aspect of exercise to some people is its help in weight loss. The more aerobic exercise you do the more calories you use, and the more fat that is burned up as energy. Any physical activity can reduce body fat and body weight by burning calories. Also, physical activity burns excess calories long after you finish exercising, by increasing your metabolic rate for several hours, and even up to 15 hours in some individuals. However, don't expect overnight changes in getting rid of extra fat deposits in certain places due to your increased metabolism, as it usually takes up to 2 months for your body's metabolism to change enough to begin using those fat deposits for energy during aerobic exercises. This is why many people who are trying to lose extra fat often get discouraged after a few weeks of exercise when they don't see quick results.

In **women**, fat is usually accumulated first in the back of the thighs, then the hips, then the midsection and finally the upper body, particularly under the arms. **Fat is usually burned up as fuel in reverse order. Thus if you want to lose a few inches from your thighs, you'll probably have to burn up excess fat in your arms, midsection and hips first.**

It takes the aerobic type of exercise mentioned earlier to help your body burn stored fat. If you do the "stop and go" type of exercise where you stop after every five minutes to rest, you will not burn stored fat. Likewise, if you eat or drink any amount of carbohydrate, including beer and sodas, shortly before or after exercising, you will not burn fat but will use up the food you ate for energy. Conversely, if you don't want to lose weight when exercising, you should eat some amount of carbohydrate before or after exercise.

After your metabolic rate has changed and you begin burning stored fat properly, your body will begin to normalize at an ideal weight as long as you eat sensibly. You may even be able to splurge once in a while enroute to your ideal weight without gaining extra weight back.

Food intake and physical activity must be kept in balance. It is **not** impossible for anyone to lose weight, including fat deposits that just don't seem to go away. They will go away if you give them time **and** effort. And it is important to always eat nutritionally to be sure your body's glands and organs have the nutrients needed to help your body function properly and to utilize food and energy for proper metabolism. You may want to take a moderate potency multivitamin/mineral supplement to be **sure** you have the proper nutritional levels for optimal metabolism.

Calories Burned by Various Activities

Activities (Averages are for a 150 lb. person)	Calories used per hour
Light	
Lying down or sleeping	80
Sitting or standing still	100
Driving an automobile	120
Rebounding slowly (mini-trampoline)	150
Domestic work (light)	180
Moderate	
Bicycling (5½ mph)	210
Walking (2½ mph)	210
Gardening	220
Golf, lawn mowing	250
Bowling	270
Swimming (¼ mph)	300
Dancing, volleyball, rollerskating	330
Vigorous housework	350

| Calisthenics | 360 |
| Wood chopping or sawing | 400 |

Vigorous
Tennis, bicycling (10 mph)	420
Skiing (10 mph), handball, rebounding, jogging	600
Basketball, jumping rope, dancing (fast)	630
Running (10 mph)	900

(You may burn up many more or fewer calories than those shown, depending upon how vigorously you perform the activity and upon your own size: The larger you are, the more calories you'll burn. Remember that the average person burns up to twice as many calories as normal for several hours following vigorous exercise.)

Exercises for Healthy Eyes

Good food creates a good blood stream, but only exercise can bring that blood stream where it is needed. Attached to your eyeballs are six fine, silk-like little muscles that can be exercised and strengthened like all other muscles of the body. Simple eye drills, which take only a few minutes a day, can greatly improve the looks and function of the eyes. Here are two simple eye drills to keep your eyes young:

(1) Turn your head from side to side as if saying an emphatic no. Do this ten times.

(2) Hold your index finger or a pencil about ten inches away from your eyes. Look at its tip, then into the distance. Do this ten times.

Do these two simple eye drills every day; do them especially when you are using your eyes intensely for close work or for reading, and your eyes will serve you better.

How to Relax Tired Eyes

Palming is the best way to relax tired eyes. Sit in front of a calendar or a picture. Look at it. Now, gently, close your eyes and cover them with your cupped palms. Be sure not to press on the eyelids. Rest your arms. Relax. Let go. Breathe deeply and slowly thirty, forty, fifty times. As you relax, your covered eyes will see only gray-black, and as you gradually let go of all tension, your eyes will see a deep, dark black. Then open your eyes. Look at the calendar or picture again. You will see it more and more clearly the more you relax. Your eyes and your whole face will lose their tension whenever you palm. Do it often.

Eating and Exercise

Anyone who exercises has to be concerned about diet. You can't feed a horse junk food and expect it to win the Kentucky Derby.

You're going to be making small changes in your body — and

big changes in your self-esteem — with your exercise program. Complement the other changes by thinking about some simple changes in your eating habits. You don't need tremendous changes in your diet; even little ones will help your over-all improvement program. For most people, the best diets are based on whole grain breads and cereals, potatoes, beans, fresh fruits and vegetables, fish, chicken, lean meat and low-fat dairy products.

Nutrition for Activity

The active life necessary to build and maintain a youthful body requires a complete nutritious base. While many nutrients, including fiber, are supplied by fresh fruits, vegetables, nuts, seeds and whole grains, vigorous exercise creates a special demand for the water-soluble B-complex and C vitamins which must be replaced daily. Also essential are Vitamin E and an adequate supply of iron, calcium, magnesium and potassium.

These nutrients play an essential role in transporting oxygen through the bloodstream to rejuvenate and repair aging cells and tissue. If you feel you are not obtaining an adequate supply from natural foods, supplements may be helpful.

The B-complex vitamins provide intricately related benefits and should all be taken together each day. The best natural sources are whole grains, wheat germ, brewer's yeast and sunflower and sesame seeds. Without an adequate supply of Vitamin B-1 (thiamin), B-2 (riboflavin) and B-3 (niacin), our bodies cannot transform natural foods into muscular energy. Vitamin B-6 (pyridoxine) helps protect against cholesterol deposits and is vital in the production of hemoglobin, the substance used by red blood cells to carry oxygen. B-12 (cyanocobalamin) is essential for tissue production and in the development of oxygen-bearing red blood cells.

An abundant supply of Vitamin C (ascorbic acid) is absolutely necessary for maintaining and rebuilding muscles and body tissue. People who fail to get enough vitamin C in natural foods may require supplements, preferably in time-release capsules combined with bioflavonoids.

Vitamin E, an antioxidant, plays a triple role in exercise nutrition. By boosting tissue oxygenation, Vitamin E creates a decided improvement in muscle performance capacity. It combines with oxygen to prevent the rupture of red blood cells, and is a powerful aid to the circulation.

Among the minerals essential to athletic performance, iron stands out for its ability to improve the quality of oxygen-bearing blood and for increasing the body's overall resistance to stress. Among other essential minerals, calcium, magnesium and potassium help in building bones and in preventing muscle cramps and osteoporosis. Calcium is essential for the absorption of Vitamin B-12. If calcium supplements are used, they should ideally also contain folic acid and Vitamin D.

While sound nutrition and a positive attitude are indispensable factors in any health-building program, we must never forget that youth IS activity. Thus, regardless of what you may have read or heard, good health, new youth and long life are not attainable without a daily program of holistic total-body exercise.

Make A Commitment

Once you start being more active, you can bet that you'll never stop. You'll get too much good out of it and enjoy the results too much to give them up. Anyone who sincerely follows such a program can expect to begin functioning like a much younger person — and to burn off surplus fat, reduce blood pressure, improve heart and lung capacity, retard aging and develop flexibility, energy and stamina.

And the results in your morale, in your self-esteem and in your determination can be spectacular.

We're asking you to take only small steps toward finding new skills — to live better, to be healthier, to handle stress better, to have a better attitude toward life and work; all in all, to feel better, look better and like yourself better.

To be able to share a better life with your family; to be able to do more things on the job and at home; to make you stronger in case of a physical or emotional problem; to give you more spirit to avoid depression. We're sure you'll agree these are all worthwhile goals and rewards.

You don't have to make a limitless commitment to physical fitness. You don't have to go all out — eat nothing but organically grown foods and run 10 miles a day. The thought that you have to do all of that would surely turn you away from the entire idea. Don't let it.

Don't refuse to do something just because you can't do everything.

Don't avoid improvement just because you cannot attain perfection.

Do what you can with whatever you can. That's all we ask.

Make up your mind to begin an exercise program **NOW** and stay with it. It may not be easy — especially at the start. But as you begin to feel better, look better and enjoy a new zest for life, you will be rewarded many times over for your effort.

Exercise has also been found to be the most effective and quickest way to boost the spirits. In fact, just 10 minutes of jogging can double the body's production of a certain hormone, norepine-phrine, that is responsible for alleviating depression and lifting the spirits. And its effect is long-lasting, too. Other chemicals are released in the brain called enkephalins that produce a natural high when exercising. Exercise is a **POSITIVE** addiction that everyone should include as part of their lifestyle.

BENEFITS AND TECHNIQUES
OF DEEP BREATHING

Good breathing techniques can:
— sharpen a dull mind
— soothe you into dreamland if you have trouble falling asleep
— perk you up in the morning if you wake up groggy
— control anger or fear
— relax from the effects of stress
— reduce tension
— improve digestion
— and more

Increasing the amount of air you can exhale after taking a breath may even help protect you from a heart attack. By changing your breathing patterns you can calm yourself and even change your mental state.

Probably the best breathing technique or breathing exercise is **deep breathing.**

Begin by breathing in slowly and evenly through your nostrils. In the first few sessions, keep your fingertips lightly on your abdomen and see how deep down into the abdomen you can breathe. Feel how your abdomen expands, then your rib cage, then your entire lungs.

To exhale, simply reverse the process, again breathing through your nostrils slowly and evenly. Finish the breath by gently contract-ing the abdomen and expelling the last of the stale air.

Don't strain. Never breathe beyond your capacity, trying to force air into your lungs. Just breathe rhythmically and easily. And try to make your inhalation and exhalation the same length. Do this by using a slow mental count to three for the length of your inhale and exhale. As your breathing capacity improves, you can work up to a higher count.

When should you do deep breathing?

The next time you lose your temper. Instead of counting to 10, breathe to three! The same goes for the next time you feel tired, tense, or bored. Just take three or four deep breaths — and then notice your livelier, calmer mood.

Other great times for deep breathing are in the morning before you get out of bed and in the evening as you lie in bed before sleep. In the morning, it can give you a lift; in the evening, it can settle you gently into sleep.

How long should you deep breathe? For as long as is comfortable. But a minute or so of deep breathing should be the minimum for best results — results beyond relaxation and calm.

Regular practice of deep breathing exercises improves the oxygen capacity of your lungs thus helping to prevent heart attacks.

When you're laid up in bed with the flu or recovering from an operation, deep breathing probably is the best exercise you can do. It can promote good circulation and thus help to prevent clots from forming.

Deep breathing can speed up your blood flow — not as much as a jog or bike ride of course, but still noticeably.

So if you want a calmer mind and a more relaxed body, take a few deep breaths, or if you want natural deep breathing, try some aerobic exercises.

WHY DO WE EAT?

The fundamental purpose of eating is to replenish the chemical elements composing the cells and tissues of our body with appropriate nutrients. Cells and tissues include our blood, organs, glands and all other functioning systems. Nourishing food provides the materials needed for your body's building and repair. It also provides regulators that enable the body to function properly. We need to continually replenish our bodies with nourishment. This is a basic law of nature.

Water, air, sunshine, and our food should provide that nourishment. Unfortunately, because our bodies seem to be able to take a lot of punishment, we can survive for years on food that is destructive to the body but appealing to our appetite and palate, **until** we finally become sick.

It only takes a little knowledge, common sense, will power and motivation to live and eat correctly so that we can attain optimum health and happiness.

THE CONSTITUENTS OF FOOD

Food provides us with proteins, fats, carbohydrates, vitamins, minerals and fiber.

Protein

Protein is important for many bodily functions. Muscle tissue as well as connective tissue throughout the body is strengthened by protein. The health of hair, skin and nails also depends on protein, as do enzyme and hormone production. Protein is made up of amino acids, which are necessary to build body cells. When protein is broken down through digestion, ammonia is formed. People who eat excessive protein or those with kidney damage may develop a strong ammonia-like body odor. Also with excess protein, the kidneys are unable to excrete all of the uric acid formed from protein metabolism. It may then accumulate in the tissues and joints, and then crystalize, producing toxicity and giving rise to the symptoms of gout. The more water you drink the easier it will be for the kidneys to flush the uric acid out of the body. With plenty of water flushing the kidneys, you can also prevent stones from forming in the kidney and bladder.

Fats

There are three natural types of fat—
1. Saturated fats from animal and some plant sources (coconut and palm oil). These fats are usually solid at room temperature.
2. Unsaturated fats from plants.
3. Monounsaturated fats from plants.
Hydrogenated fats are a fourth form of fat that is usually found in shortenings and margarine. These are similar to saturated fats in their effects on the body. Overconsumption of animal fat and hydrogenated fat can cause a severe overload on your body's metabolism.

Fats supply twice the amount of calories that either protein or carbohydrates provide, and therefore are the most concentrated source of energy. (Carbohydrates are the **healthiest** source of energy, however). Fats are needed in the diet to act as carriers of the fat-soluble Vitamins, A,D,E, and K. Fat is also used to convert beta carotene from green, yellow and orange vegetables to Vitamin A in the body. Deposits of fat surround and protect various organs as well as provide a layer of insulation on our bodies to prevent extreme temperature changes. Essential fatty acids from unsaturated fats are necessary for the body to manufacture certain hormones and are also important for the health of the skin, hair and mucous membranes. Unsaturated fats have a tendency to lower blood cholesterol levels, while saturated fats tend to raise cholesterol levels. Monounsaturated fats do not affect the cholesterol levels. Olive oil and peanut oil are examples of monounsaturated fats.

Carbohydrates

Carbohydrates are the body's most efficient and easily digestible source of energy. All foods contain carbohydrates, except meat. Carbohydrates are of two types, refined and unrefined. Refined carbohydrates include all types of sugars and sweeteners, as well as processed grain flours (white flour) that have had the fiber and germ, as well as some vitamins and minerals, removed from them. Unrefined carbohydrates are also called complex carbohydrates. The sugars and starches of fruits, vegetables, whole grains, nuts, seeds and legumes are included in this group.

Sugar And Other Refined Carbohydrates

Sugars are absorbed into the bloodstream so quickly that the pancreas releases massive amounts of insulin to control them. The body is then flooded with insulin and causes the blood sugar to drop off sharply, creating a craving for sugar, exhaustion, and sometimes dizziness, nervousness and headaches. This excess insulin will then readily convert these refined carbohydrates to fat whenever our body cannot use them for energy. Too much sugar also robs the body of B complex vitamins that are needed to metabolize it. Keep sugar consumption of any kind to an absolute minimum. One good way to do this is by gradually reducing the amount of sweeteners called for in recipes and by substituting fructose or fruit juice.

Sugars are high in calories and low on nutrition. All refined grains are also high in calories and low on nutrition, except for containing a small amount of protein. White flour products, as well as white rice, are mostly starch, with most of the B vitamins, Vitamin E, fiber and minerals removed.

Be careful to watch for hidden sugars in many foods such as sweetened canned fruit, catsup, and hundreds of others.

Complex Carbohydrates

Complex carbohydrates take much longer to digest than refined carbohydrates. Because they digest slowly they help the pancreas keep the blood sugar level stable. This prevents numerous health problems from occuring including hypoglycemia, headaches, dizziness and even diabetic tendencies. The need for insulin injections has even been reduced for many people. The complex carbohydrates release glucose slowly into the bloodstream so that energy reaches the brain, nervous system and muscle tissue in steady amounts. The brain functions much better mentally and physically when energy is released slowly. Increasing your consumption of complex carbohydrates also helps you increase your dietary fiber intake.

Fiber — Benefits For Your Diet

If you eat plenty of fiber, or roughage, you shouldn't need laxatives such as mineral oil or chemical preparations. Sufficient dietary fiber should be part of your daily nutrition. You shouldn't think of it as something to use only when you have symptoms of constipation, but rather think of it as a **preventative** to constipation and a number of other illnesses.

Fiber affects the consistency and bulk of digested material in the intestine. Since fiber holds water, stools produced by a high fiber diet tend to be bulkier and softer and pass more quickly and more easily through the intestines. This in turn means less strain and pressure on the bowels and blood vessels. Thus fiber helps to eliminate constipation and hemorrhoids.

If you do feel the need for a laxative, there are gentle herb-based products that can help you. Harsher laxatives can actually weaken your intestinal muscles and you could eventually become dependent on them.

Getting sufficient water and fiber in your diet and exercising the abdominal muscles through stretching, situps, toe-touching, etc. can help to tone the intestines to enable them to do their part in elimination. All of these factors will minimize strain and help prevent hemorrhoids, diverticular disease, colon cancer, varicose veins and other health problems.

Many people who need additional fiber rely solely on wheat bran. If you do use wheat bran, it is best to eat it cooked or soaked to neutralize the phytic acid that can bind minerals and make them unusable. There are many other dietary fibers that are gentler and more beneficial. These include oat bran and the fibers found in fruits and vegetables — gums, pectins and storage polysaccharides (hemicelluloses). These are known as **soluble fibers.** Soluble fibers form gels in the intestinal tract and moderate the absorption of nutrients (including sugars) in the small intestine at a more gradual speed, thus preventing steep rises in blood sugar. This type of fiber also tends to lower serum cholesterol levels.

A balance of **all** fibers — soluble and insoluble — will keep food moving through the intestines at the proper rate. By causing more frequent bowel movements, the fiber will absorb toxic metals, chemicals, bad bacteria, toxins and cancerous substances that may be produced in the intestine from improper digestion and elimination. It will remove impacted fecal matter from intestinal walls and cavities, and will regulate the absorption of sugars, fat and cholesterol.

Fiber has additional benefits for people trying to control their weight. Because fiber expands with moisture, it satisfies a person's hunger more quickly. It has also been postulated that less fat and cholesterol are absorbed by those on a diet with sufficient fiber.

Be sure to drink plenty of water to keep the fiber moist in your intestines so that it moves smoothly, quickly and thus without irritation. Drinking two to three glasses of lukewarm water upon arising will not only provide moisture for the intestines but will also help the bowels function with regularity. Don't just add fiber such as wheat bran to a poor diet and think your problems are solved. You must also be sure to eat foods that are **naturally** high in fiber. By regularly eating high-fiber foods, you will gradually come to prefer them. (Note: Oat bran is easier on the intestinal lining than wheat bran. It is also lower in phytic acid than wheat bran.)

The following charts list the amount of dietary fiber found in some common foods. Note the substantial difference in the fiber levels of complex and refined carboydrates:

Dietary Fiber Content of Foods

Refined Carbohydrates	Serving Size (★½ cup cooked unless otherwise indicated)	Total Fiber (grams)	Soluble Fiber (grams	Insoluble Fiber (grams)
Spaghetti	1	0.8	.02	0.8
White bread	1 slice	0.8	0.03	0.8
White rice	★	0.5	0	0.5
Complex Carbohydrates				
Bran 100% cereal	★	10.0	0.3	9.7
Whole grain bread	1 slice	2.7	0.08	2.6
Rye wafers	3	2.3	0.06	2.2
Oats, whole	★	1.6	0.5	1.1
Brown rice	★	1.3	0	1.3
Legumes				
Kidney beans	★	4.5	0.5	4.0
Pinto beans	★	3.0	0.3	2.7

Complex Carbohydrates	Serving Size (raw)	Total Fiber (grams)	Soluble Fiber (grams)	Insoluble Fiber (grams)
Vegetable				
Potatoes	1 small	3.8	2.2	1.6
Broccoli	*	2.6	1.6	1.0
Carrots	*	2.2	1.5	0.7
Tomatoes	*	2.0	0.6	1.4
Cauliflower	½ cup raw	0.9	0.3	0.6
Lettuce	*	0.5	0.2	0.3
Nuts				
Almonds	10	1.0		
Peanuts	10	1.0		
Fruits				
Apple	1 small	3.9	2.3	1.6
Pear	1 small	2.5	0.6	1.9
Banana	½	1.3	0.9	0.4

Meats, milk products, eggs and fats and oils are not listed in this food fiber survey because they are virtually devoid of fiber content.

Vitamins

Vitamins are substances found in food, that when taken into the body become constituents of enzymes necessary for activating thousands of body functions. Individual needs for vitamins vary widely, depending on inherited characteristics, biochemical individuality, environmental factors, and the type of foods you eat. Vitamins are either water-soluble or fat-soluble.

Fat-Soluble Vitamins

The fat-soluble vitamins are A,D,E and K and are measured in international units (IUs). Their absorption and assimilation are aided by the oils and fats in foods. Therefore if you take supplements of any of these vitamins, you should take them with meals that have significant amounts of fat and oils. You also need adequate bile secretion to use the fat-soluble vitamins properly. Excess fat-soluble vitamins are stored in the liver for use as needed. The range of requirements for these vitamins vary, but each person has a maximum safe dose of each fat-soluble vitamin. Since these vitamins do build up in the body, you can accumulate toxic levels if high doses are taken for a long time. If you do supplement with fat-soluble vitamins, especially vitamin A, watch carefully for any signs of toxicity.

Water-Soluble Vitamins

The water-soluble vitamins are all those except A,D,E and K, and are measured in micrograms and milligrams. Your body cannot store water-soluble vitamins. You need a fresh supply daily. Since they are water-soluble, these vitamins leave the body through perspiration and urination. If you get more than you need of a water-soluble vitamin in your diet, perspiration and urine carry away the excess. It is generally safe to take extra doses of water-soluble vitamins, although the kidneys may need to work somewhat harder excreting them. Cooking destroys water-soluble vitamins. This is a good reason to lightly steam, rather than boil your vegetables. With either method, we suggest that you save the water you used. It is rich in nutrients and you can then either drink it or use it in another dish.

Minerals

Minerals found in food are also necesary to activate many biological processes in the body. As with vitamins, mineral needs of individuals can vary considerably. Many vitamins work properly only in the presence of certain minerals. Of the seventeen "essential" minerals, seven are macro-minerals (those that you need in significant amounts) and the others are considered trace minerals (only small amounts are needed).

Toxic Minerals (Metals)

There are also several minerals that are detrimental to the human body. Those are sometimes referred to as toxic metals and include lead, mercury, cadmium, aluminum and others. They usually get into our bodies as a result of pollution from various sources. The sea, the soil, the air and even our water supply have all been found to contain some concentration of these toxins.

Lead and cadmium are common in industrial and auto emissions, paint, ink, rubber products, cigarette smoke, etc. Mercury is often found in significant amounts in polluted waters and thus ends up in our fish supply along with other chemicals. Aluminum poisoning, now thought to be the cause of Alzheimer's Disease (senility), is sometimes a result of cooking with aluminum cookware.

At even low concentrations, these substances can have toxic effects when they are taken into your body. Be careful of the sources of your food and water. Hair analysis, an inexpensive service offered by many health professionals, can help determine the presence of toxic levels of these minerals. Vitamin C, Selenium and many other nutrients can help to draw these toxins from the body.

THE IMPORTANCE OF GOOD NUTRITION

Nutrition can mean the study of diet and health. It also refers to nourishment of the body through the digestion and assimilation of nutrients.

Good nutrition is necessary to help all the body's organs function correctly. It will increase physical and mental strength and resistance to disease. Eating whole unprocessed foods and being aware of proper food choices are the most important factors in good nutrition. Whole foods can be an alternative to drugs and medicine by helping the body to produce its own antibodies to fight infection, by giving the body natural protection against pollution, and by reducing the harmful effects of stress on the body.

First and foremost you should choose foods as close to their natural state as possible. With whole foods you will regain your natural taste for real foods that are less sweet, less salty and which contain no artificial colors and flavors and no preservatives. Processed foods are incomplete and do not contain the nutrients and micronutrients that work synergistically to aid in the utilization of foods. Not only is the quantity of nutrients reduced but even the quality of the nutrients that are left is lowered by extreme processing techniques. If we eat foods that have had their nutrients partially destroyed, our whole body suffers. The more processed and devitalized foods you eat, the more vitamins and minerals your body will need. It will demand nourishment. This demand for food often leads to overconsumption and weight gain.

Your mental attitude can also suffer from poor nutrition. Stress situations can then begin to cause more extreme reactions, such as unusual irritability or moodiness. This can cause relationships with your family or friends to deteriorate. You may even realize that you are not performing as well at your job as you can. Good nutrition is important for all aspects of your life. We cannot control all influences on how we look and feel, but nutrition is one we can. It is never too late to start a good nutritional program.

Proper nutrition should become as routine for you as getting up in the morning. **You** must be in charge of your nutrition, rather than your emotions or your appetite, or even fancy packages.

Many people eat when they are anxious, sad, lonely, or bored. Not only do these people end up eating junk food, but they also have a tendency to become obese. Soon this becomes a cycle. They get depressed because they are overweight and then eat because they are depressed. For your health, your appearance, and for your family, take charge of your nutrition. No one else will do it for you, but by reading this book, you will be well on your way to being in control.

Encourage your children at an early age to take responsibilities in the kitchen—both for food preparation and cleaning up. It is a great help to busy mothers and fathers to have every member of the family comfortable in the kitchen and able and willing to do all chores. It will also be a good opportunity to discuss and explain good nutrition to your entire family.

Four important factors for a good nutritional program are:

1. Eat at least three well-balanced meals per day. Several well-known university studies (including the University of Iowa Breakfast Studies) have shown that those who eat breakfast tend to be more alert, productive and efficient than those who go to work or school on an empty stomach.

2. Avoid overcooking your food.

3. Avoid fast foods and convenience foods.

4. Avoid dieting and skipping meals.

With whole foods you will regain your natural taste for real foods that are less sweet, less salty and which contain no artificial colors and flavors and no preservatives.

Whole foods may be an alternative to drugs and medicine by helping the body to produce its own antibodies to fight infection, by giving the body natural protection against pollution, and by reducing the harmful effects of stress on the body.

NUTRITION AND YOUR CHILDREN

The standards of good nutrition and good health in general hold true for both children and adults. The effects of violating these standards during the growing years of children are serious and can affect them in their later life. Studies have shown that babies allowed to become fat have a very high chance of remaining fat the rest of their lives. The importance of diet during these growing years is particularly significant. Inadequate nutrition can cause a brilliant and attractive child to become physically and mentally less capable. Children will be more apt to enjoy their school work and have an easier time learning if given good nutrition.

Maximum nutrition is important not only during the main growing years, but all the way through adolescence. Everything eaten needs to be nutritious to maintain good health. A multiple vitamin/mineral supplement may also be beneficial.

It is now generally recognized that defects in our physical structure can be due largely to deficient food quality. Children need to be persuaded against any diet featuring refined products and high fat foods, and encouraged to eat a diet rich in whole foods such as grains, seeds, legumes, nuts, fresh fruits and vegetables.

Never keep junk foods in the house. For snacks, carrot and apple slices and other nutritious alternatives will help children learn good eating habits. Just be creative and imaginative and the children will love it. By eliminating undesirable foods gradually, especially sugar and sweets, you can help children change to a better diet. A good diet for your child (and for you as well) will not only limit, and eventually eliminate, harmful foods, but will also build resistance to sickness and disease at the same time.

Once you have made the commitment to good nutrition, the easiest and most effective way to introduce this to your family is to encourage them to develop a respect for good nutritious foods and eating habits. It is up to the parents to counter the effects of advertising on TV from food manufacturers and fast food restaurants. Parents should also work together through your PTA and your childrens' school administrators to serve the most nutritious food they possibly can and in particular to get them to stop serving junk foods and heavily sugared foods. For assistance in this endeavor you can write to the National Nutritional Foods Association, P.O. Box 2089, Carlsbad, California 92008-0350 for a packet of information that can help to improve school lunch programs.

Your entire family can enjoy the benefits of good nutrition!

DIETARY GUIDELINES OF THE UNITED STATES BY THE SENATE SELECT COMMITTEE ON NUTRITION AND HUMAN NEEDS

Following is a statement by Senator George McGovern, past Chairman of the United States Select Committee on Nutrition and Human Needs.

"The simple fact is that our diets have changed radically in the last 50 years, with great and often very harmful effects on our health. These dietary changes represent as great a threat to public health as smoking. Too much fat and too much sugar or salt can be, and are, linked directly to heart disease, cancer, obesity and stroke, among other killer diseases. In all six of the ten leading causes of death in the United States have been linked to our diet."

The following U.S. Government dietary guidelines are based on thorough and exhaustive findings by the U.S. Senate Select Committee on Nutrition and Human Needs.

1. EAT A VARIETY OF FOODS. Assure yourself an adequate diet. The greater the variety the less likely you are to develop either a deficiency or excess of any nutrient, whether it be protein, carbohydrates, fats, fiber, vitamins or minerals. Variety also reduces your likelihood of being exposed to excessive amounts of contaminants.

2. MAINTAIN IDEAL WEIGHT. If you are overweight, your chances of developing some chronic disorders are increased. Obesity is associated with high blood pressure, increased levels of blood fats (triglycerides) and cholesterol, diabetes, heart attacks and strokes. To lose weight you must take in fewer calories than you burn. You can either select foods that contain fewer calories, or increase your activity levels—or both. Eat less fat and fatty foods, less sugar and sweets, and avoid too much alcohol. If you need to lose weight, do so gradually. To maintain your weight, all you need to do is take in as many calories as your body uses.

3. AVOID TOO MUCH FAT, SATURATED FAT, AND CHOLES-TEROL. Individuals eating diets high in these foods have greater risk of heart attack than people eating low-fat, low-cholesterol diets. Eating too much saturated fat will increase blood cholesterol levels in most people. To avoid too much fat and cholesterol:

a. Choose dry peas, beans, fish, poultry, low fat dairy products or lean meat as your protein sources.

b. Moderate your use of eggs and organ meats.

c. Limit your intake of butter, cream, hydrogenated margarines, shortenings, coconut oil and foods made from such products.

d. Broil, bake or steam rather than fry.

e. Read labels carefully to determine both amount and types of fat contained in foods.

4. EAT FOODS WITH ADEQUATE STARCH AND FIBER. Carbo-hydrates contain half the calories per ounce as fats. Complex car-bohydrate foods such as whole grain breads and cereals, fruits and vegetables, beans, peas and nuts are good sources of fiber, starch, protein and other essential nutrients. Eating more foods high in fiber tends to reduce symptoms of constipation, diverticulosis, and some types of "irritable bowel." There is also concern that low-fiber diets might increase the risk of colon cancer.

5. AVOID TOO MUCH SUGAR. A major health hazard from eating too much sugar is tooth decay. The risk of tooth decay is increased not only by the sugar in the sugar bowl, but also by the sugars and syrups in jams, jellies, candies, cookies, soft drinks, cakes, and pies, as well as sugars found in products such as breakfast cereals, catsup, flavored milks and ice cream. Frequently the ingredient label will provide a clue to the amount of sugar in a product. To avoid excessive sugar consumption use less of all sugars including white, brown and raw sugar, honey and syrup, and eat less of the foods mentioned above. Select fresh fruits or fruits canned without sugar or syrup. Read food labels for sugar content. Sucrose, glu-cose, maltose, dextrose, lactose, fructose, and syrups are all sugars. Of these, fructose probably causes the least amount of stress on your metabolic functions, since it is metabolized slower. How often you eat sugar is as important as how much sugar you eat.

6. AVOID TOO MUCH SODIUM. Sodium appears in many pro-cessed foods, condiments, sauces, snacks and many other foods. People take in much more sodium than what they need. The major health hazard is high blood pressure, though sodium is only one factor affecting it. (Obesity also plays a major role.) To reduce your consumption of sodium, eat less table salt, limit your intake of salty foods, learn to enjoy unsalted flavors of food, and read food labels for salt content.

7. IF YOU DRINK ALCOHOL, DO SO IN MODERATION. Alcoholic beverages tend to be high in calories and low in other nutrients. Vitamin and mineral deficiencies occur commonly in heavy drinkers —in part, because of poor food intake and also because alcohol alters the absorption and use of some essential nutrients.

'Other Effects And Alternatives'

Sustained or excessive alcohol consumption by pregnant women has caused birth defects. The child's body will contain the same concentration of alcohol as the mother's but is not developed enough to metabolize it. Mental as well as physical defects will result and can affect the child for the rest of its life. Even after the child is born and is breast feeding, the mother should not drink alcohol since her milk will contain nearly as much alcohol as her blood.

Heavy drinking may also cause a variety of serious conditions, such as cirrhosis of the liver and some neurological disorders. Alcohol can also kill brain cells. Cancer of the throat and neck is much more common in people who drink and smoke than in people who don't. If you drink alcohol, do so in moderation. Those who are heavy drinkers must first recognize and admit that they have a problem before they can get their habit under control. You can help these people through your example and friendship.

There are many excellent nonalcoholic beverages available now that are good alternatives to beer, wine, champagne, etc. Several good nonalcoholic beers include Kingsbury, Birell and Texas Select. Recently, several de-alcoholized wines have been introduced on the market. They undergo the full fermentation process and then have their alcohol removed with a technique that requires no heat. The resultant beverage tastes exactly like wine but has less than ½% alcohol. Other good wine alternatives include white and red grape juice, sparkling apple juice and flavored mineral water. Most of the beverages we've mentioned can be obtained from either health food stores, specialty stores or liquor stores. In some areas, you may also be able to find wines that have been grown by natural methods — no chemical pesticides or insecticides used on the grapes.

Preservatives and additives in alcoholic beverages are another reason to minimize your consumption. Several different forms of the preservative sulfur dioxide can cause allergic reactions in some people. There are many other additives, colorings and flavorings added to beer and wine. For a complete list, read 'Chemical Additives in Booze' researched by the Center for Science in the Public Interest, Box 14176, Washington, D.C. 20044.

Dietary Goals of the United States suggest that protein make up 12% of the calories in a healthy person's diet. Fats should constitute no more than 30% of the calories you eat. (American Health and Nutrition suggests 20% as a much healthier figure.) No more than 10% should be saturated fat from animal sources (excluding fish). The Dietary Goals recommend that 48% of the diet consist of complex carbohydrates and naturally occurring sugars. It is also suggested that consumption of all sugars and sweeteners be reduced to 10% or less of your diet.

The Senate Select Committee cited findings which show that dramatic improvements could be made in the health of most Americans. The figures indicated that if Americans ate less sugar, salt, fat, and processed foods and more whole grains, fresh fruits and vegetables, the benefits that could result include:

- 90% elimination of **Allergies** due to food
- 80% reduction in incidence of **Obesity**
- 75% reduction in **Osteoporosis** (Bone disease)
- 50% less afflictions of **Arthritis**
- 50% of **Diabetes** cases avoided or improved
- 50% reduction in incidence, severity and expenditures for **Dental Problems**
- 50% reduction in **Infant Mortality**
- 33% reduction in **Alcoholism**
- 25% fewer **Digestive Problems**
- 20% reduction in deaths and acute conditions of **Kidney** and **Urinary Problems**
- 20% reduction of **Respiratory** and **Infectious Ailments**
- 20% reduction of **Cancer**
- 20% fewer people blind or with corrective lenses **(Eyesight)**

CONCLUSIONS AND FINDINGS
Select Committee on Nutrition And Human Needs
Of The United States Senate

1. Americans lack understanding of the consequences of nutrition related diseases.

2. Millions of Americans are actually sick with diet related illnesses. Six of the leading causes of death in the United States are connected to diet.

3. We do know that millions of Americans are failing to realize their full potential because they do not have a proper diet.

4. The American public is eating blindly. Medical schools have underemphasized nutrition with the result that the typical physical examination does not involve thorough nutritional evaluation or counseling. The starkest evidence of medical neglect of nutrition is the prevalence of malnutrition in hospitals.

5. The American people know more about what their cars need than what their own bodies need. The result is an American public tempted by unhealthy food and which is therefore a physically unhealthy nation.

6. There is much greater recognition today of the fact that the kinds and amounts of food and liquor we consume and the style of living of our sedentary society are major contributing factors in the development of chronic illness.

7. One in three men and one in six women in the United States can be expected to die of heart disease or stroke before the age of 70.

8. Twenty-five million Americans suffer from high blood pressure and five million are afflicted by diabetes. These diseases are directly related to the over-consumption of certain foods.

9. Millions of Americans are not receiving the nutrients they need. For example, significant numbers of children are deficient in iron.

10. The strength of the nation is based upon the health of its people.

11. Overeating by Americans is likely to make them obese, give them high blood pressure, and induce heart disease, diabetes and cancer. In short, it can decrease their life expectancy. We face the tragedy of anemic children failing in school and repeating that pattern of failure throughout their shortened lives.

12. Better health, a longer active lifespan, and greater satisfaction from work, family, and leisure time are among the benefits to be obtained from improved diets and nutrition. Most of all, the health problems underlying the leading causes of death in the U.S. could be modified by improvements in the diet.

"Health is almost always undermined by slow and unseen causes acting for a long time; the most important of these causes is improper diet."

—Dr. E.V. McCollum, John Hopkins Hospital

The U.S. Food and Nutrition Board, the National Academy of Science and the USDA agree that you may not even be getting the minimum recommended daily allowances (RDA) of nutrients that your body requires unless you consume from the four food groups at least:

- Four or more servings of fruits and vegetables.
- Four or more servings of bread and cereals (whole grains).
- Two to four servings of dairy products, tofu (from soybeans) or other foods high in calcium and protein, such as tahini (sesame seed butter).
- Two or more servings of beans, peas, fish, eggs, or meat.

Following these recommendations and using cooking methods that preserve the maximum amount of nutrients should provide you with sufficient fiber, protein, vitamins, minerals, carbohydrates and fats. As much as possible avoid the 5th food group — fats, sweets and alcohol.

Today, over 100 million Americans are suffering from one or more of these serious health problems, many of which are a result of poor nutritional habits:

Heart Disease	26 Million
Arthritis	16 Million
Diabetes	10 Million
Ulcers	17 Million
Osteoporosis (Weakened Bones)	4 Million
Allergies	40 Million
Obesity	55 Million
High Blood Pressure	23 Million

At the present rate, 55 million Americans may get cancer during their lifetimes. Many types of cancer have also now been related to diet.

"I saw few die of hunger; of eating, a hundred thousand."
— *Benjamin Franklin*

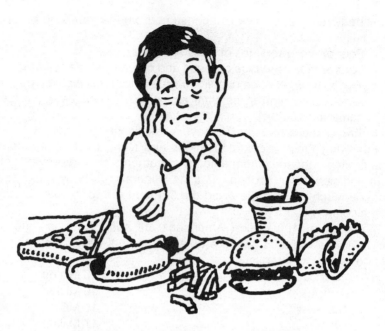

"A regular burger, fries, and soda amount to a meal that falls short in every nutrient studied."

—Dr. Paul Chance, Rutgers University

"The typical McDonald's meal does not give you much nutrition and is typical of the diet that raises the cholesterol level and leads to heart disease."

—Dr. Jean Mayer, Harvard University

Simple Food Preparation Changes For Better Nutrition

- *Broil, bake,* or *poach* meat, chicken, or fish rather than fry.
- *Season* foods with curry powder, garlic, onions, dry mustard powder, oregano, basil, and other herbs instead of butter and salt.
- *Reduce sugar and fats* in cookie, cake, pie, and pudding recipes.
- *Add less oil or butter* to soups, sauces, and casseroles.
- Saute foods in small amounts of *vegetable oil* rather than frying.
- Baste meat or poultry with *wine, fruit juice, onions* or *garlic* rather than fat.
- Cream soups with *flour, vegetable oil, and skim milk* instead of whole milk or cream.

- *Add less mayonnaise* to egg, chicken, potato, tuna, or Waldorf salads (mix mayonnaise with plain, low-fat yogurt to further reduce fat calories).
- Season sweet dishes with *cinnamon, nutmeg, and ginger* to enhance sweetness and reduce sugar.
- *Steam* vegetables lightly rather than boil to retain vitamins, minerals, and enzymes.

Examples of Simple Menu Substitutions

- *whole wheat* for white bread
- *brown rice* for white rice
- *skim or low-fat milk* for whole milk
- *tuna packed in water* for tuna packed in oil
- *low-fat cottage cheese* for regular cottage cheese
- *canned fruit packed in juice* rather than syrup
- *frozen yogurt* for ice cream; and
- *whole milk* for artificial coffee creamers.

When using recipes, be aware of how you can change the recipe to make it more healthful using some of the suggestions above. Don't feel that you have to strictly follow a recipe to make it taste good.

VEGETABLES

Fresh vegetables are much more nutritious than canned or frozen. Canned vegetables are very devitalized and are usually high in salt and other additives. The closer to the raw state that you can eat vegetables, the more nutrition and texture you can enjoy. Eating plenty of raw vegetables will give you many vitamins, minerals, and fiber, as well as enzymes that act as catalysts in digesting, assimilating, and utilizing your foods. If you do cook your vegetables, you should lightly steam or stir-fry rather than boil them. Steam cooking your foods will retain more flavor, more nutrients and more color. 4 to 10 minutes is sufficient for most vegetables. You should save the water, and either drink it or use it somewhere else in your meal, as it contains many nutrients. Vegetables should never be cooked to the point of losing their crispness. When you cook a dish that includes vegetables, be careful not to overcook. The peels and skins of vegetables and fruits contain a significant amount of nutrients. Just wash them rather than peeling.

Try to choose those vegetables with the highest amount of nutrients. Include plenty of dark green and yellow leafy vegetables such as romaine lettuce and broccoli, as well as starch-type vegetables like squash and carrots. Lightly steaming some vegetables, especially carrots, can make some of their nutrients more available.

An easy way to eat lots of raw vegetables is by creating colorful and healthful fresh salads. But don't drown your salad in fancy brand name dressings. There are many delicious homemade dressing recipes that are not only healthier but cost less. Even your waistline will benefit.

FRUITS

Fruits too should be eaten fresh whenever possible. If you buy canned fruits, be sure to choose only fruit packed in water or juice. Even though fruit juices contain high concentrations of their own natural sugars, they are not as nutritious as whole fruits. Pasteurizing juices destroys vital enzymes and vitamins. It is much easier to control your blood sugar levels with **whole** fruits just as it is with other **whole** foods. As with vegetables, you should try to obtain fruits that have little or no chemicals applied to them. Home dried fruit is a fairly good alternative to fresh fruit since it is not processed like canned fruit. It is usually sunripened or dehydrated at low temperatures. If you buy dried fruit do not buy the type that is preserved with sulphur dioxide. For snacks, fruits satisfy a craving for sweets and the urge to chew while providing useful nutrients.

Fresh fruit makes a good dessert. Try pureeing blueberries and serving them on sliced fresh peaches. You can have the satisfaction of preparing a creative, tasty, nutritious, eye-pleasing and appealing dessert.

Since they are body-cleansers, fruits are also especially good to "**break**-the-nights-**fast**."

Cleaning Fruits And Vegetables

For those people who do not have easy availability to fruits and vegetables that have been grown without chemicals, we suggest rinsing or bathing them in either a vinegar or lemon juice solution. This will remove not only some of the chemical residue but also dirt, bugs, etc. A salt solution will also help to remove bugs. A good vegetable bristle brush is also useful in cleaning your vegetables. By doing these things you can avoid peeling your food and losing the abundance of fiber and other nutrients in the peel.

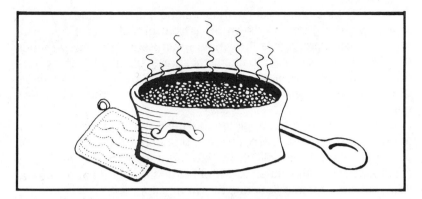

WHOLE GRAINS

Whole grains consist of brown rice,wheat, oats, rye, corn, millet, buckwheat, barley, etc. Avoid, as much as possible, any white flour products, white rice, white pasta, degermed corn meal and other processed grains. As with vegetables, use the lowest heat possible when you cook grains. It is helpful to soak grains overnight or up to 24 hours (until soft and just beginning to sprout), then cook at a low temperature (130°-150°) until soft and tender. You could use either a crockpot, oven, or electric skillet for easier temperature control, or use a double boiler to cook the grains. Steaming the grains is also a good way to cook them. Another interesting way to eat grains is to grow them as sprouts for a couple of days and then use raw on salads, or lightly cook in soups, casseroles, hot cereals, etc.

Grains that have been processed into white flour are devoid of many nutrients. They no longer contain fiber (bran), germ or oil. Both the bran and germ contain many vitamins and minerals including natural Vitamin E. What remains after processing is a devitalized product that, when mixed with moisture in the intestine, becomes like paste. It is easy to see why so many people have intestinal problems.

While chewing all food is important for good digestion, chewing grains is probably more important. Try to chew grains at least fifty times to maximize the benefit of the digestive enzymes in the saliva and give the rest of your digestive system an easier task.

A side benefit of sufficient chewing is that this strengthens the teeth and gums, and can reduce periodontal (gum) disease.

Many people do not think of grains as having much protein. Instead they think of grains as starches. This is probably true for **processed** grains, since they have had a certain amount of protein, fiber, vitamins and minerals removed. Whole grains contain a substantial amount of protein. Other sources of protein, such as beans and peas or animal proteins, should be added to your daily diet to complement the grain protein, thus making it more usable.

If you can't grind your own flour from grains, visit a health or natural food store where the whole grain flours are usually much fresher and less exposed to chemical sprays, etc. than those a commercial supermarket may carry. You will also be able to find whole grain breads that are much more nutritious than those on supermarket shelves.

If you are allergic to the gluten in wheat, there are several excellent grains that contain very little or no gluten. Brown rice and oats are good alternatives. Millet, buckwheat and corn also have only small amounts. Substitutes for whole wheat flour in recipes are oat flour, soy flour, potato flour and brown rice flour.

Savory Rye, Brown Rice and Kidney Bean Casserole

This unusual casserole combines the flavor of rye with the delicate flavors of the herbs and vegetables. Add salad and a leafy green vegetable for a light meal.

Cooked tender:
  ½ cup whole rye
  ½ cup brown rice
  (Any grains may be used)
  6 tbsp. kidney beans or other beans or peas
1 stalk celery, chopped
1 cup tomatoes, chopped fresh
  (or canned)
½ tsp. dill seeds, ground
¼ tsp. sage
2 tbsp. or less tamari soy sauce
1 egg, beaten
½ cup grated cheese

1. Combine all of the ingredients EXCEPT the grated cheese.
2. Turn the mixture into an oiled casserole.
3. Bake at 350°F for 45 minutes, until firm, sprinkling the grated cheese over the top during the last 10 minutes of baking.

4 Portions

1 portion = approximately 10 grams of usable (complete) protein *(approximately 20 to 25% of daily protein needs)* Taken from *Recipes For A Small Planet*

LEGUMES (BEANS AND PEAS)

Legumes are also rich in complex carbohydrates and have an even higher protein content than grains. Some legumes are soybeans, peanuts, dried peas, lentils, mung, kidney, azuki, black, lima, navy, pinto and red beans. Though they have often been referred to as the "poor man's" diet, they should perhaps be called the "healthy person's" diet. In many countries, except for parts of Western Europe and America, beans and peas are one of the most highly valued and important ingredients in the diet. Compared to meat, legumes have many more health promoting properties. Legumes have significant protein, fiber, vitamins, and minerals, and contain no cholesterol. In fact, only animal products contain cholesterol. Tofu and tempeh are soybean products that are good protein foods. Tempeh is a cultured whole-soy product that when fresh has a taste resembling fresh peas, mushrooms or fish. Tofu is the protein of soybeans that is formed into a cheese-like cake with a custard-like texture, delicate flavor and creamy white color. Tofu can be baked, sauteed, scrambled, made into dips, dressings, desserts, burgers or added to any number of dishes.

Many experiments have actually shown legumes to reduce blood fats and decrease arteriosclerosis, and yet many people shy away from legumes because they find them difficult to digest. Legumes can cause intestinal gas if not prepared properly. Anyone not used to eating beans and dried peas should start by eating only a small amount. Soaking legumes overnight permits the enzymes in the bean to breakdown the starches into sugars. You should then pour out the soak water and rinse the beans. This will help to further eliminate gas-causing properties. Very thorough cooking for up to an hour further breaks down the starches. The popular tofu has already undergone extensive cooking preparations and will cause little gas. Tempeh, being a cultured product, has also had its starches broken down through enzyme action. If you soak the legumes overnight or longer, and then grow them as sprouts for one, two, or even more days, they do not need as much cooking, since the sprouting action breaks down the starches to sugars. Give beans a chance. They are a bargain in cost and nutrition.

NUTS AND SEEDS

Nuts and seeds are a significant source of protein. Nuts, grains, and legumes are all seeds, but foods most commonly referred to as seeds are pumpkin, sunflower, sesame, and flax. Nuts are high in beneficial oils and therefore are high-calorie foods. Seeds have less oils, but are more commonly used as a source of cooking oils since most are less expensive. Seeds and nuts can be used in casseroles, burgers, sauces, desserts and many other dishes. Because they are so high in calories, use them as a complement to other foods. As with grains and legumes, the digestion of seeds and nuts can be improved by soaking or sprouting. Many nuts and seeds are sold as "butters," just like the familiar peanut butter. Tahini is an excellent spread or sauce made from hulled sesame seeds. Grinding seeds into butters is a good aid to their digestion, but you should still remember that it is important to chew everything thoroughly.

SPROUTS

Sprouts are living foods. Some of the more popular are sprouts from mung and soybeans, lentils, alfalfa and wheat, though many others are very tasty, such as sunflower, cabbage and radish. Use them on salads, sandwiches, or any other dish you prepare. Cook mung and soybean sprouts at least for a short time. If you grow your own sprouts, be sure to buy untreated seeds. Health and natural food stores are the best place to find them. They also carry products for you to use when sprouting. An easy method of sprouting is:

1. First rinse the seeds, using thin cloth or cheese cloth as a screen.

2. Soak them in a jar for six to eight hours, or overnight in lukewarm water, or only a few hours in warm water.

3. Fasten a cloth over the mouth of the jar.

4. Drain this water and rinse again.

5. Set jar at 45° angle in either a dark ventilated place or just keep covered with a cloth.

6. Rinse seeds twice a day. Soybeans should be rinsed three or four times per day.

7. Sprouts should be ready to eat within two to tour days.

You may want to expose alfalfa and some other sprouts to light for the last day. This adds flavor and increases the content of chlorophyll, Vitamin C, and other vitamins that benefit the body. Sprouting increases protein content and makes the protein and starches more digestible. Sprouting grains will also neutralize the phytic acid we mentioned earlier. Since sprouts are a live food, they also contain many enzymes that promote necessary enzyme reactions in the body. Fresh vegetables too, contain these enzymes.

Try to grow as many of your own vegetables and other foods as you can. Only then can you be sure of the nutritional environment of the soil in which your foods are grown. You will also know which agricultural chemicals are used on the food you eat. The more chemicals you can avoid, the better off you will be. For all healthful foods that you can't grow yourself, we suggest you visit a health or natural food store and look for the most healthful foods you can find in your supermarkets.

DAIRY PRODUCTS

Many people cannot digest dairy products. This is often the result of the lack of an enzyme called lactase that digests lactose or milk sugar. Raw milk, which has not had its natural enzymes destroyed, is easier to digest, as is goat's milk, but should only be purchased if it is processed by a certified dairy. Cultured products such as yogurt, sour cream, buttermilk and cheese are all easier to digest since they contain large amounts of helpful bacteria and enzymes that break down the lactose. Some people feel that dairy products are mucous forming. This may be a result of pasteurization that not only kills certain enzymes but also heats the protein molecules to an extent that causes them to be more difficult to digest. Homogenizing milk also changes the structure of the fat molecules thus creating more confusion for your digestive system. For those who can't digest milk products, lactase enzyme supplements are available that can help, and there are vegetable alternatives such as soy milk, almond or other nut milk.

PROTEIN ALTERNATIVES IN THE DIET

Meat, poultry, dairy products, fish and eggs are usually considered "the protein foods." Fish, eggs and yogurt are probably the most healthful of these proteins. Eggs have the most complete and utilizable complement of amino acids, fish has the lowest fat content, and lowfat yogurt is possibly the most easily digestible. There are many other foods that contain substantial amounts of protein. Beans and peas have a high percentage of protein, with soybeans being higher than even meat. Nuts, seeds and grains also contain substantial quantities of protein. When a person gets some foods of both of these categories in their diet, the combination creates high quality protein. Grains and legumes are the best partners in creating good protein since their amino acid contents complement each other well. The best ratio of eating them in your daily diet is 2 portions of grains to 1 portion of legumes. For example, if you eat ½ cup grain with ¼ cup lentils you will have made both foods a complete high quality protein. Of course if you eat more than that amount of either food, you will still get some protein from the extra portion along with all the other nutrients it contains. By eating even small amounts of eggs, dairy products and other animal protein foods, you will also utilize the proteins of grains, legumes, nuts and seeds more efficiently.

Many vegetables and fruits also contain small amounts of protein. These proteins too are utilized by the body when included with other foods in the diet.

There are many vegetable protein alternatives to the traditional protein foods. These are often more economical sources of protein than meat, especially when prepared at home. Grain, legume, nut and seed combinations can be made or purchased in many forms.

Many health problems can be prevented by eating more vegetable proteins in the diet especially as an alternative to eating meat and other high-fat foods. We suggest and recommend that you experiment with these non-meat proteins.

Some people think that without eating plenty of meat they won't get enough protein in their diet. Adults should get from 45 to 55 grams of protein every day. This recommended allowance could be met with the following non-meat foods eaten in one day:

	Grams of Protein
1 cup soybeans, cooked or 6 oz. tofu	15
1 egg	6
½ cup milk or yogurt	4
1½ oz. cheese or 2 oz. of fish	11
4 servings fruits and vegetables	8
4 servings whole grain breads and cereals	9
TOTAL	53

SHOULD YOU DECREASE YOUR MEAT CONSUMPTION?

Even though meat is a good source of complete protein and our ancestors ate it for hundreds if not thousands of years, there is now enough scientific data to establish the reality and seriousness of possible detrimental effects of meat eating. Statistics show that people who eat little or no meat are slimmer, healthier and live longer.

Most Americans eat much more meat than they need to meet their protein requirements, and consequently their fat needs as well, thus contributing to overweight problems. It is agreed that meat eating is a major factor in the disease and mortality rate in the United States. It is actually harder to get a nutritionally well-balanced meal with meat than without meat, for several reasons.

First and most importantly, meat has too much fat. Even if you trim the fat off the meats, it may still have a high fat content. It is best not to use the liquified fat from cooked meat for gravies and sauces. It has been suggested that it is the high fat content of a diet, especially one based on meat, that is the principle cause of breast cancer and colon cancer, as well as the many other problems associated with the blood system and heart.

When cooking roasts, stews, etc., you can chill and lift off the hardened fat as a way of reducing your fat consumption. It is also a good idea to brown meats and poultry and then pour off the fat before continuing with a recipe. Or you can cook meats and poultry on a rack that allows the fat to drain off.

Secondly, meat has no fiber to keep it moving through your intestines. This problem may be even worse than those associated with the fat content. Because there is no fiber in meat, meat takes two to three times as long as other foods to go through your intestines. During this time it begins to ferment and putrefy, producing many types of gases and acids. These cause bad breath, foul-odored stools and a general decrease in energy.

Meat is one of the hardest foods to digest, taking five to six hours as opposed to just one half to one hour for fruit, two hours for vegetables, three hours for grains and somewhat longer for most other protein foods.

Because of meat's long passage time through the intestines and the resulting putrefaction, it has been directly connected to colitis, diverticulosis, and colon cancer. This long intestinal time is also a major cause of constipation. Another problem is that of hemorrhoids, caused partially from constipation and more directly from large, dry stools, which put strain on tiny blood vessels, causing them to burst.

The third nutritional problem associated with meat is the calcium-phosphorous ratio. Because meat is so high in phosphorous compared to its calcium content, it upsets the nutrient balance, and calcium is leeched from the bones. This also occurs because a high protein diet causes an increase in the urinary excretion of calcium.

Excess meat also causes uric acid to build up in the body. This can lead to kidney disorders because the kidneys can become enlarged and inflamed while trying to process the excess nitrogen, a by-product of protein breakdown. This is particularly true for those who eat a lot of meat. It can also happen on other very high protein diets.

Meat is a difficult food to digest, assimilate and eliminate, and therefore can put a greater wear on the various organs and systems of your body.

There are also the possibilities of salmonellosis and trichinosis which can come from contamination and undercooking, respectively. Be sure to cook pork thoroughly to prevent trichinosis and keep all meat refrigerated.

Discussed so far have only been the physical and nutritional problems associated with meat eating. Most of us could probably come up with other reasons for limiting the amount of meat we eat, but we will stay with the nutritional aspects of meat eating in this book.

All of this is not to say you shouldn't eat meat, but you should be selective in the type of meat you do eat, and try to limit the amount you eat as much as possible — for the best possible state of health.

Let's put some type of order to the types of meat you should choose, going from the **least** favorable to the **more** favorable for your health.

1. Any ground meat, which includes hamburger, sausage, all processed meats — hot dogs, cold cuts,etc. Ground meat spoils faster outside of and inside of your body. You can grind meat yourself and use it while still fresh or freeze for later use. Processed meats have not only been ground but contain higher amounts of fats, and many contain potentially harmful preservatives to keep them from spoiling fast.

2. Smoked and charcoaled meats — these meats contain carcinogenic chemicals; charcoal is very toxic. We suggest using wood chips for grilling, or at least grilling on foil as opposed to open flame.

3. Bacon or other high fat meats.

4. Whole pork or beef — roasts, chops, steaks, etc.

5. Poultry — skin removed.

6. Fish.

Any meat raised free of chemicals is obviously preferred.

With reduced meat consumption, you can still get plenty of protein from eating cheese, yogurt, eggs, fish and combinations of beans, soy products, peas, grains, nuts and seeds. All animal products are complete proteins. Vegetable products contain incomplete proteins. To get complete proteins from vegetable products you should eat legumes (beans or peas) including tofu and tempeh, with grains, nuts, or seeds, or include a small amount of animal protein to complement these foods. These various proteins do not all need to be combined in the same meal but you should eat a variety in the same day for the best combination of protein amino acids.

Special Hints For Those Who Eat No Animal Foods

In addition to being sure to get complementary protein from all possible plant sources — fruits, vegetables, grains, legumes, nuts and seeds — vegetarians who do not eat milk products, eggs or meat should consume plenty of green leafy vegetables for needed iron, folic acid and other vitamins; increase their caloric intake by eating more of what they do eat; be sure to get some form of vitamin B-12 in their diet either from a food that is fortified with it, or B-12 supplement, or foods such as tempeh, spirulina, kelp, bee pollen, comfrey, etc.

USING FATS AND OILS

Avoid frying vegetables and other foods as much as you can. Lightly sauteeing with low heat still retains many nutrients, but frying devitalizes food. Frying also adds fats to food, making them more difficult to digest. This extends the digestion time and uses up more energy in the process. Eating fried foods is probably one of the main causes of weight gain as well as being the possible cause of other health problems. Frying with animal fat (lard) or shortening (partially hydrogenated oils and fats), is very conducive to weight gain and to an increase in cholesterol.

If you fry with vegetable oils you should use those with high heat resistance — olive, peanut or sesame. The more unsaturated the oils, such as corn, safflower, or sunflower, the more unstable the oil becomes, and thus the more rancid and carcinogenic it can become. **All** of these oils should be cold pressed (preferably mechanically pressed) and as unrefined and unfiltered as possible. The vegetable oils you do use should be obtained in small quantities, then kept tightly sealed in the refrigerator. One or two capsules of vitamin E in a bottle of vegetable oil will help preserve the oil. You should definitely not reuse these oils. The lower the heat you use, the more nutritious will be your food. This applies to baking as well as frying. The highly unsaturated oils are best used with foods that don't require cooking.

SALT AND OTHER CONDIMENTS

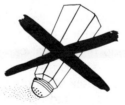

One thing that **can't** be taken with a grain of salt these days is the amount of salt in the American diet. That's because salt contains sodium. Sodium has been directly linked to high blood pressure and other health problems. There is mounting evidence that it may contribute to strokes and other cardiovascular diseases as well.

Excess sodium upsets the delicate sodium/potassium fluid balance in your body. This causes several problems, first of which is upsetting the pressure between cells, as water is forced from inside the cells to the outside. For many people, salt causes edema, or fluid retention. Edema symptoms include puffiness and swelling of the ankles and face. Edema is often accompanied by high blood pressure. This fluid imbalance causes thirst, and often is a cause of dry skin and loss of skin elasticity. Salt can also cause rashes on the body and can interfere with circulation in general. Excess salt can be an irritant to your stomach and can interfere with your digestive processes. Because it disguises the food you eat from your taste buds and stomach, your body is confused about which digestive enzymes to produce. Condiments of all types will cause this problem.

(Many condiments such as vinegar, black and red pepper, horse-radish, mustard and even garlic and hot onions can cause irritation to the delicate cell lining of your stomach and interfere with diges-tion. Garlic and onions do have some medicinal effects on the body, but are best eaten cooked rather than raw, to lessen their irritation. Vinegar has been known to kill red blood cells at the same rate as alcohol. If you use these condiments at all use only very small amounts. The only kind of vinegar you should use is real apple cider vinegar.)

Our total salt requirement is less than ½ teaspoon per day. This is equivalent to 2500 mg. of salt or 2000 mg. of sodium. "Excess" sodium is almost any amount more than you get in a normal diet of unprocessed foods that have no salt added. For example, green leafy vegetables and dairy products are naturally high in sodium. Most cheeses and butter, however, have even **more** salt added to them. Fortunately, low-salt cheese and butter are now available to consumers.

Celery and other vegetables also contain small amounts of sodium naturally. These form the basis for very flavorful powdered vegetable seasonings and broths that can be found in health and natural food stores. These stores also have other low sodium sea-sonings, as well as large varieties of herbs and spices for flavoring your meals. A salt substitute called potassium chloride is available as well.

You can learn to enjoy these new methods of flavoring food as much as you did salt. When you leave out the salt and eat your foods with their own flavor, you will know the true delicious taste of the food you are eating, not a disguised taste.

Some people add salt to their food for iodine, a necessary min-eral. However, adequate iodine can be obtained by eating seafood or sea vegetables. Mushrooms, garlic and wheat germ are other whole foods that contain small amounts of iodine. You can also get iodine in a multiple vitamin-mineral supplement or in a kelp tablet available in health and natural food stores.

Most Americans consume 10 to 20 times as much salt as recommended. Salt is present in thousands of foods, and even in some beverages and soft drinks. Most baking soda and baking powder also contains sodium, as does MSG (monosodium glutamate). Monosodium glutamate is used in a large variety of prepared foods. It is most widely used in the oriental foods served in many restaurants. Many people experience headaches, dizziness and other ill-health symptoms after eating meals in oriental restaurants. Some studies have also found monosodium glutamate to be carcinogenic (cancer causing). In some of the better Chinese food restaurants you can ask for meals prepared without MSG. Never be afraid to ask!

Salt is an acquired taste. We are not born with it. People who eat a lot of salt when young gradually become physiologically addicted to it. Those who have become addicted to the taste of salt usually feel they need to add salt to their food even if it already has salt in it. As with sugar, if you **want** to cut down on adding salt to your foods, just don't buy it. **Rather than eating what you like, learn to like what is good for you.**

WHY WORRY ABOUT CAFFEINE?

Caffeine can cause periods of sleeplessness, irritation and anxiety in doses of either 200 to 300 mg. at one time or 600 mg. throughout the day. Many people develop other symptoms including headaches, heartburn, ringing in the ears, rapid breathing, depression, diarrhea, etc. Even babies who are nursing develop sleep problems if the mother is a coffee drinker. Coffee can also seriously deplete your body of nutrients, especially the B Complex and C vitamins, iron and potassium. It is the caffeine in coffee that is responsible for this. Regular coffee is usually around 2½ to 3 percent caffeine. Even the small amount of caffeine still remaining in decaffeinated coffee, approximately ½ percent, can cause some of the same effects as 3 percent caffeine, only to a lesser degree.

Caffeine causes overproduction of insulin resulting in low blood sugar and loss of energy. So when you drink coffee your body is fighting itself, at first being stimulated from the caffeine and then losing energy as the overproduction of insulin causes the blood sugar to drop. This insulin overproduction by the pancreas will gradually weaken the pancreas. According to Harvard researchers, coffee may cause more than 50 percent of cancer of the pancreas in the United States. (This deadly form of cancer takes the lives of

20,000 Americans annually). An earlier study showed a correlation between coffee and cancer of the bladder. Caffeine holds a real hazard to young children since it may cause damage to brain and central nervous system development. Another problem associated with coffee drinking is the damage it does to the linings of your stomach, especially the higher acid, higher caffeine coffees. The digestive and eliminative systems are victims of coffee consumption as well. Both diarrhea and constipation can result. Blood pressure problems are also common with heavy coffee drinkers.

Many people feel they can get rid of their drag and sluggishness each morning and each day by drinking coffee. In reality it is the coffee and the violation of the other laws and principles of good health that cause the sluggish feeling.

Perhaps the most detrimental aspect of coffee consumption, whether caffeinated or decaffeinated, is that it contains residues of some of the most toxic insecticides, herbicides and other chemicals used on plants in the world today. Some of these chemicals have even been banned in the United States and sold to countries that produce most of the coffee in the world. Many of these chemicals have been proven to be hazardous and harmful to your health, even carcinogenic.

Even the process of decaffeinating coffee uses dangerous chemicals, the residue of which remains in the coffee. Some coffees do use a water decaffeinating process. This is not harmful, although the original chemicals used in growing the coffee beans remain.

Some health and natural food stores today carry organically grown coffees — coffee grown without harmful chemicals. These particular varieties are naturally only 1 percent caffeine.

While most people know of the caffeine in coffee and cola drinks, many are not aware of the caffeine that comes in other drinks, as well as in nonprescription drugs. Again, the bottom line is to read the labels. **Know what is in any product before you buy it.**

How can you know if you are addicted to caffeine? Stop using it for two or three days. Addiction will then manifest itself in the following withdrawal symptoms: headache (coming around eighteen hours after the last consumption of caffeine), drowsiness, much yawning, nervousness, lethargy, lack of concentration, runny nose and diarrhea. These symptoms can last for at least two weeks. Clearing all caffeine from the system will probably take several days.

Following are some suggestions that may help you cut down on your coffee consumption.
 (1) If you feel you have the "will power" to give it up all at one time, go ahead and give it a try.
 (2) Simple, progressive reduction in the amount you consume

is a good way to cut down. If you can't go without the morning "perk-me-up" at least start by cutting out the "social" coffee at your work breaks, lunch hour, etc. When you're successful at cutting out one cup per day, try for two.

(3) If you have a strong desire for coffee, try making it weak and drink only one cup or less.

(4) Get someone else at work and/or home to cut back with you. A supportive partner always helps. You will enjoy exploring other beverage alternatives together. Try the large variety of hot and cold beverages that are caffeine free. These range from grain based "coffee substitutes" to herbal teas, decaffeinated coffee, etc.

Soon, you'll be able to avoid the energy ups and downs associated with caffeine consumption. You'll be able to fall asleep faster and sleep more soundly. Thus, you'll feel less groggy in the morning and won't feel the urge to have that morning perk-me-up. To help diminish the desire and need for coffee, it is very important to follow healthy ways of eating and living.

OTHER CAFFEINE PRODUCTS

Caffeinated teas, colas and some other soft drinks, and even chocolate, contain caffeine and can cause the same problems as coffee. But they have additional problems of their own.

Dark tea has large amounts of tannic acid, which has been shown to cause cancer. Colas contain large amounts of other acids that are harmful and destructive to the blood, digestive system and overall health of your body. Some other soft drinks contain these acids as well. The acid raises your blood stream to harmful acid ph levels. This can gradually lead to sickness and disease.

Another danger associated with dark teas results from the sizable amount of sugar many people add to them to improve their taste. And of course soft drinks have too much sugar to start with. There are natural colas and soft drinks available without caffeine but they too should be consumed infrequently because of their high content of sweetener. However, many are now being sweetened with aspartame, a sweetener that is hundreds of times sweeter than sugar. Therefore, very little is needed to sweeten the product. Studies are still being done to verify its complete safety.

A good alternative to chocolate is carob. Carob is a very nutritious food with a natural sweetness. It is also low in fat and contains a significant amount of protein.

ARTIFICIAL COLORINGS, FLAVORINGS AND OTHER CHEMICAL ADDITIVES

Anything artificial in your food is going to do you more harm than good. Chemicals in your food can cause rashes, hyperactivity, allergies, blood pressure problems and nervousness.

Always read food labels carefully. Ingredients are listed in order, by the weight of the quantity of each. Any ingredients that sound like chemicals usually are chemicals. You should avoid these, as well as foods containing sugars, salt or fats as one of the major ingredients.

Does anyone really think that Jello, Kool-aid, Tang and thousands of other so called food products on the market (more appropriately — nonfoods) are nourishing and good for our health?

Examples of delicacies from the chemistry lab:

TANG Breakfast drink—sugar, citric acid, calcium phosphates, modified starches, potassium citrate, cellulose gum, Vitamin C, hydrogenated coconut oil, artificial flavor, artificial color, Vitamin A palmitate, BHA.

LIPTON Cup A Soup—BHA, propyl gallate, citric acid, corn syrup, monosodium glutamate, hydrogenated vegetable oil, modified corn starch.

JELLO Dessert—sugar, adipic acid, disodium phosphate, fumaric acid, artificial color, artificial flavor—imitation cherry flavor is made up of eugenol, cinnamic aldehyde, anisyl acetate, anisic aldehyde, ethyl oenanthate, benzyl acetate, vanillin, aldehyde C 16, ethyl butyrate, totylaidehyde, benzealdehyde, alcohol.

READ LABELS!

As one example of how you can make your own alternatives to these foods, we suggest that instead of buying gelatin mix, you purchase pure unflavored gelatin and mix it with pure fruit juice, fruits and nuts. Or you can go to a good natural food store and buy a pure natural gelatin dessert mix—no chemicals. You can also purchase agar-agar, a natural powdered gelatinous plant thickener that you can just mix with water.

Summary of Foods That Can Be Detrimental To Good Health

1. White Flour Products and Refined Grains

white rice	macaroni	doughnuts
white bread	biscuits	pie crusts
crackers	cakes	cookies
spaghetti		

2. White Sugar and Other Highly Sweetened Products

pastries	beer	pudding
pie	candy	cake
sodas	jelly	doughnuts
	milkshake	ice cream

3. Foods High in Fat

hamburgers	lard	oily snacks
french fries	shortening	fried and deep
fatty meats	margarine	fried foods

4. Harsh Spices and Condiments

horseradish	vinegar (especially	raw hot onion
mustard	distilled)	and garlic
	red pepper	

5. Foods High In Salt

canned soups	snacks	seasoning high
packaged sauces	condiments	in salt or MSG
		(monosodium
		glutamate)

6. Products With Caffeine

coffee	sodas
black teas	chocolate

7. Products Containing Chemical Additives

DIGESTION AND FOOD COMBINING

Digestive enzymes are produced by several different organs in the body. Without proper digestive enzymes we would be unable to digest, absorb and assimilate the foods we eat. We've all heard the saying "You are what you eat." More appropriate would be "You are what you eat, digest, and assimilate." Your digestion begins by chewing food as thoroughly as possible, in a relaxed mental atmosphere, so that your digestive enzymes are secreted in adequate amounts and at the right times to enable your body to have an easier task with digestion. Indigestion often results from no chewing food properly. Setting your fork or spoon down between mouthfuls is a good way to help you get into the habit of chewing your food thoroughly.

Another major cause of indigestion is improper food combining. This often results in poor utilization of the foods you eat. Other important causes of digestive problems include eating under stress, overeating, eating late at night, eating while fatigued or while you have strong emotions. Snacking between meals also upsets the digestive process still going on from the previous meal. The absorption of vitamins, minerals, protein, fat and carbohydrates could all be impaired. This in turn can lead to many nutrition-related illnesses.

We should also keep the consumption of liquids at mealtime to a minimum so as not to dilute the digestive juices of the stomach. Consumption of alcohol and sodas with meals also slows digestion and can cause fermentation and gas. Alcohol causes the protein digesting enzyme pepsin to separate from the food mass in the stomach.

The better your digestion is, the shorter the time that food remains in the stomach and intestines. Due to the warm temperatures in the stomach, the longer it takes for food digestion, and the greater the chances that putrefaction of proteins, fermentation of sugars, and rancidity of fats and oils will occur.

Many people tend to eat more food at their meals than they can digest easily. This is especially harmful when proteins, refined carbohydrates and fats are all eaten at the same meal. Refined carbohydrates include sugar and white flour products such as pastries, pies, cakes, sodas, beer, white bread, macaroni, spaghetti, fruit, fruit juices, candy, and all other sweets and sweeteners. Even whole grain (complex carbohydrates) desserts should not be eaten with proteins or fats unless they are very low in sugar content.

Protein foods, as well as fats, can take up to five hours to digest in the stomach before moving to the small intestine where digestion is completed. During this time, the sugars of the refined carbohydrates react with bacteria and the warm temperature in the stomach and begin to ferment and cause gas. This gas buildup is partially responsible for the uncomfortable full feeling some people have after meals. Belching and burping can also result. When gas accumulates in the upper intestine after meals, bloating, cramping and even pain can occur.

The more gas in the intestine, the more difficult it is for the nutrients to be absorbed there. The movement of food through the intestines is also slowed by pockets of gas, allowing toxins produced from the fermentation and putrefaction to be partially reabsorbed into the blood. Digestive enzyme supplements that contain hydrochloride, pepsin, pancreatin and bile can be helpful in preventing a buildup of gas by speeding up the digestive process. Large meals, poor food combining, and all the other causes of indigestion, are reasons why we may benefit with digestive supplements. A digestive enzyme supplement should be taken with your meal for maximum benefit.

Another important benefit of good digestion and sufficient fiber in the diet, and thus better movement through the intestinal tract, is that the colon (intestine) will stay healthy. Problems such as constipation, colitis, diverticulosis, diverticulitis, and cancer of the colon can all be minimized.

Some other irritants to the digestive tract include caffeine and other stimulants, harsh spices, drugs, and pesticides and herbicides in the food supply. These irritants can cause allergic reactions in the intestine and allow crude or undigested proteins to be absorbed back into the bloodstream. These in turn cause allergic reactions related to other parts of the body.

Special attention to all your nutritional habits as well as getting plenty of exercise are important to good intestinal health and bowel care. Everyone should take a brisk walk after meals to increase the oxygen levels in the blood. This usually helps digestion and prevents the sluggish feeling often associated with large meals. Eating more than your body can digest easily can dull the senses as well as drain your energy. The saying "Eat breakfast like a king, lunch like a prince, and dinner like a pauper" is very fitting for your best digestion. Your digestion secretions slow down as the day goes on.

Heartburn

Heartburn is yet another prevalent problem associated with digestion. It gets its name from the feeling of acid irritation at the top of the stomach, which lies slightly below the heart. We have been led to believe by antacid advertising that heartburn is a result of too much acid in the stomach. Actually the process leading to heartburn often begins with a lack of hydrochloric acid. This can slow the process of digestion to a point where the enzyme bile is sent back from the duodenum (that part of the intestinal tract immediately below the stomach) back into the stomach. Bile is alkaline and since the stomach tries to maintain an acid environment, it secretes hydrochloric acid. Heartburn results from this overstimulation of acid. If this process of irritation to the stomach by bile and acid occurs often, the stomach lining is weakened and ulcers may begin to form. A supplement of hydrochloride with the meal, as well as proper food combining, may prevent heartburn.

Alcohol and coffee beverages can also add acidity and increase the likelihood of heartburn. Since high fat foods are hard to digest they stay in the stomach longer and cause more acid to be produced which can also lead to heartburn.

One more thing about heartburn. After a heavy meal, you may feel drowsy. Resist the temptation to lie down. It is best to remain upright either sitting or standing. When one lies down, the stomach contents can back up and cause heartburn or other distress. It is probably okay to lay down for a **few** minutes however.

Digestive Enzymes

The enzyme **Ptyalin** is found in saliva. The more you chew your food, the more ptyalin is produced. This is especially important for digesting complex carbohydrates and other starches. Ptyalin is an alkaline enzyme that is inactivated by acidity. Therefore eating acid foods with carbohydrates neutralizes the action of ptyalin and slows the digestion of carbohydrates and starches. Likewise, acidity of the mouth caused by bacteria reacting on food particles left between the teeth will also partially neutralize ptyalin. If you eat carbohydrates first in your meal, the ptyalin will continue to work in the stomach until foods with a higher protein content increase hydrochloric acid secretions that stop starch digestion.

Most people usually eat proteins and complex carbohydrates at the same meal. This is why it is so important to chew your food thoroughly. The starches need to be almost completely digested in your mouth since their digestion is stopped by hydrochloric acid secretions when protein is eaten.

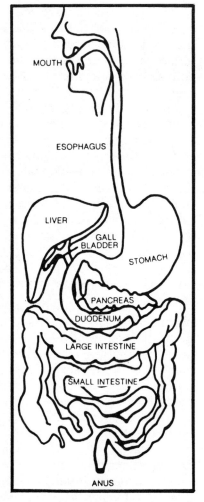

Because protein does need sufficient acid for its digestion, it may be wise to eat proteins first so the stomach acid is not diluted by other types of foods.

Although it is impractical for most people, one good method of food combining would be to eat your complex carbohydrates (beans, grains, nuts, seeds, starchy vegetables) with leafy and flower vegetables at one meal and more concentrated proteins with leafy and flower vegetables at the next meal. This will allow the starches to be digested not only in the mouth, but also in the stomach, and thus prevent fermentation.

Hydrochloric Acid (HCL) is a secretion from the stomach that helps to begin the breakdown and digestion of proteins. This gastric juice assures an acid environment in the stomach until protein digestion is completed. Hydrochloric acid also helps to keep undesirable bacteria under control in the digestive system. Low levels of HCL have been associated with cancer. The stomach also produces another enzyme called **Pepsin** that aids in the digestion of protein.

Bile is formed in the liver from cholesterol. The bile is stored in the gall bladder and secreted into the small intestine to aid in fat digestion and absorption. Bile breaks down the fat molecules. When bile contains high concentrations of cholesterol, gall stones begin to form. This is another reason for keeping the liver, gall bladder, and intestines in good health. **Pancreatic enzymes** are produced by the pancreas and secreted into the small intestine to complete the breakdown of proteins, carbohydrates and fats.

Summary of Good Eating Habits
For Better Digestion

1. Chew your food thoroughly and slowly.
2. Don't overeat, eat only when you are hungry, and avoid late night meals.
3. Combine your foods properly for best digestion.
4. Rest after eating.
5. Allow four to five hours between meals or as long as you can.
6. Eat food at room temperature as much as possible. Both hot and cold foods have negative effects on body functions. You should consume food **and** water at moderate temperatures.
7. Eat in pleasant surroundings among pleasant people.
8. Eat a large variety of foods each day.
9. Eat raw foods whenever possible.
10. Minimize your intake of processed foods, salt, sugar, fat and chemical additives.
11. Limit consumption of condiments.
12. Avoid caffeine.

13. Read food labels.

14. Start each day with a good breakfast-even a small amount of something nutritious will be helpful.

15. Avoid fluids as you eat. Most liquids such as soup, water, soda pop, alcoholic beverages, coffee, etc. merely add to the bulk in your stomach and to a stuffed feeling.

16. Take a break before dessert, allowing time for your stomach to properly digest the main meal.

Nearly every disease of mankind springs in whole or in part from wrong eating. Most diseases have their origins in the substances taken into our body.

Following all the guidelines mentioned in this book should improve your digestion and your physical and mental health but will not assure either perfect digestion or perfect health. How close to perfect health you would like to be is up to YOU!

BENEFITS OF DISTILLED WATER

As mentioned earlier, much of the drinking water found today is contaminated with a variety of chemicals and pollutants and thus treated with chlorine as a result. The chlorine does not eliminate toxins. It merely kills bacteria and germs. There are now more than 12,000 different types of chemicals on the market today, with approximately 500 more being added each year. In one way or another, many of these chemicals find their way into our water. Today we may be drinking the residues from fertilizers, pesticides, herbicides and industrial wastes, etc. As if the above mentioned chemicals weren't enough, many of these chemicals interact to form potentially dangerous combinations, some that can have accumulated effects. Many of these combinations and accumulations of chemicals, and interaction of chemical combinations, have already been researched and implicated in various illnesses and in some cases even death. Water treatment facilities cannot eliminate many of the toxic substances.

Most people do not realize the relationship between 'drinking' water and health. Most of us only think about the quality of water if it has an unusual taste or smell, but some of the most toxic chemicals cannot be seen or tasted.

Even bottled spring water in some instances has been shown to contain pollutants. The most feasible way to insure pure drinking water is by drinking distilled water. By distilling it with your own distiller the cost ranges from only 15 to 25¢ per gallon.

The distillation process is similar to the way rain water is formed. When heat is applied to water it merely evaporates and rises into the atmosphere, is cooled and eventually falls as rain. Distilled water is water which is free of minerals and pollutants. Through the evaporation process, we have learned from nature how to purify water for today's needs.

TOXINS

Many diseases, illnesses, and ill-health symptoms are a result of toxic waste accumulations in our blood, cells and organs. Toxins can be taken into your body directly, through your skin, through the air you breathe, the liquids you drink and the foods you eat. They can be in the form of chemicals, bacteria, germs, etc. Toxins can also be produced through various chemical reactions that take place in the body. Cancerous substances can be formed from chemicals taken into the body reacting with substances natural to the body.

Just trying to metabolize pollutant chemicals, or chemical food additives taxes the body's organs. The organs may be weakened and you may feel less energy. The more of these you can avoid, the more efficiently your body will operate.

Many toxins are formed in the body as a result of improper digestion and elimination. Putrefaction of proteins, fermentation of carbohydrates, and rancidity of fats and oils cause toxins to be produced in the stomach and intestines. These can be reabsorbed into the bloodstream and then into other organs of the body. All the systems of the body can become overburdened trying to metabolize and eliminate the toxins. The more toxins you have in your body, the harder it is to eliminate them. Sufficient fiber moving through the intestines will speed up elimination and minimize the absorption of toxins.

Toxic buildup in the blood is often related to headaches, nausea, fever and a host of other problems. Your body is trying to eliminate the toxins in as many ways as it can. Body odor, breath and stools all end up with foul smells. Bad breath can also result from bacteria in the mouth reacting with food that is coating your tongue, and with food that may be lodged in your teeth and gums.

As we said earlier, it is very important to brush and floss your teeth correctly every day and also to brush your tongue to keep it clean. The gums should be gently massaged with your toothbrush, especially along the gum line. This will not only help to dislodge food particles and remove plaque but will also stimulate and strengthen the gums. Whenever you eat a meal or just a nibble, you should rinse your mouth with water to keep food particles from fermenting. As a side benefit, you will prevent tooth decay and gum disease.

Toxins that are released through the skin are the major cause of bad body odor. It is important to cleanse the entire body regularly to keep these toxins from being reabsorbed into the skin.

Toxins can cause many illnesses as the body seeks to purify itself and to maintain and restore its normal state of health. Disease can result from violent eliminative efforts and thus weaken the body even more. In many instances, illness does not suddenly happen to someone, but is a culmination of a longer period of bad habits.

When our organs, glands, and all bodily systems are well nourished, freed of toxins and other causes of ill health, our body can then begin to heal itself. The lungs, liver, kidneys, bowels and skin are organs that help with elimination. It is therefore extremely important to keep these organs in good health.

That is why daily exercise, good eating habits, drinking plenty of water, getting sufficient fiber in your diet, avoiding unhealthy foods, liquids, and other harmful substances is so important in preventing and eliminating toxins. The chlorophyll in green vegetables and wheat grass can also be helpful in neutralizing toxins.

FASTING AND CLEANSING

One effective means of overcoming minor ailments is fasting. Fasting rests your body so that it has an opportunity to "clean house." The body is self-correcting and will expel toxins and wastes more easily. The best conditions for fasting include digestive rest, fresh air, pure water, sunshine, a relaxing and beautiful environment, and freedom from stress, worry and anxiety. This will allow the body to concentrate its energies on cleansing and it will often heal itself when given these proper conditions.

Unless you are very careful of your diet, it would be beneficial to fast one day a week, even when not noticeably ill. This would allow your body the time it needs to cleanse itself of accumulations of toxins and wastes. If you feel you can't do this, then one day a week try to lengthen the time between the last meal of the day and the first meal of the next day before you "Break-fast." Drink plenty of water to help flush your body as well as to satisfy any feelings of hunger. Drinking raw vegetable juices and unsweetened fruit juices would be beneficial during a fast to help cleanse as well as nourish the body. Even a partial fast that would include just one or two foods in the diet (especially raw vegetables) would be helpful to allow the body to catch up on its work. For long fasts you should seek the advice of a healthcare professional.

There are natural intestinal aids available that will assist your body in cleansing and detoxifying, and in establishing beneficial lactobacillus, bifidus or acidophilus bacteria in the intestines. This beneficial bacteria digests the bad bacteria in your intestines, therefore it is important to have a sufficient supply. Antibiotics, and fermentation and putrefaction in the intestines, can severely reduce these bacteria. Almost everyone could benefit by using intestinal cleansing aids and acidophilus supplements. Eating yogurt that contains live bacteria, as well as eating unpasteurized fermented foods like sauerkraut, miso, tempeh, etc. can be very helpful in establishing a beneficial environment in the intestines.

The intestines of most people are coated with old fecal matter, especially of those who haven't had sufficient fiber in their diet throughout their lives. This material has become compacted over the years, much like the way waterpipes and water heaters build up layers of materials. This may also be a cause of constipation in some people. In others, the bowel lining is weakened and becomes distorted causing poor movement through the intestine.

This coating on the intestines may be trapping gases and other toxins that are partially reabsorbed into the bloodstream through the intestinal walls, causing additional problems and symptoms. The layer of matter is also blocking the absorption of nutrients into the bloodstream. That is why it is so very important to keep the intestinal tract clean. The occasional use of an intestinal cleansing aid is helpful, but above all, you must eat plenty of fiber in your diet. Fruits, vegetables, whole grains, legumes (beans and peas), nuts and seeds, etc. are all good sources.

FINDING YOUR IDEAL WEIGHT

You should try to maintain "ideal" weight.

There is no absolute standard to determine your ideal weight. There are several charts published which offer "acceptable" ranges for most adults. As there are numerous variables which affect the optimum weight for each individual, these ranges should serve as guidelines, and not rigid laws, to establish a level of ideal weight.

Weight, height and bone structure all determine *your ideal weight*. Obviously a "big boned" person can carry more weight than a "small boned" person and not be overweight. The two charts below are guideline averages and will tell you very quickly in what range *your ideal weight should fall*. Our opinion is that if people weigh 10 lbs. less than these tables, they may live longer and be even healthier.

Ideal Weight Tables

MEN

Weight in pounds (in indoor clothing — for nude weight deduct 5-7 lbs.) Height measurements are without shoes.

Height		Small	Medium	Large
Feet	Inches	Frame	Frame	Frame
5	1	112-120	118-129	126-141
5	2	115-123	121-133	129-144
5	3	118-126	124-136	132-148
5	4	121-129	127-139	135-152
5	5	124-133	130-143	138-156
5	6	128-137	134-147	142-161
5	7	132-141	138-152	147-166
5	8	136-145	142-156	151-170
5	9	140-150	146-160	155-174
5	10	144-154	150-165	159-179
5	11	148-158	154-170	164-184
6	0	152-162	158-175	168-189
6	1	156-167	162-180	173-194
6	2	160-171	167-185	178-199
6	3	164-175	172-190	182-204

WOMEN

Weight in pounds (in indoor clothing — for nude weight deduct 2-4 lbs.) Height measurements are without shoes.

Height		Small	Medium	Large
Feet	Inches	Frame	Frame	Frame
4	8	92-98	96-107	104-119
4	9	94-101	98-110	106-112
4	10	96-104	101-113	109-125
4	11	99-107	104-116	112-128
5	0	102-110	107-119	115-131
5	1	105-113	110-122	118-134
5	2	108-116	113-126	121-138
5	3	111-119	116-130	125-142
5	4	114-123	120-135	129-146
5	5	118-127	124-139	133-150
5	6	122-131	128-143	137-154
5	7	126-135	132-147	141-158
5	8	130-140	136-151	145-163
5	9	134-144	140-155	149-168
5	10	138-148	144-159	153-173

Average Calorie Intake We Should Consume

Plan your maintenance diet as carefully as you would plan a reducing diet. To know the number of calories you should eat, multiply your ideal weight by:

- 12, if you're sedentary or inactive.
- 15, if moderately active.
- 17, if you're very active.

For example, if your ideal weight is 130 lbs. and you're moderately active, you would need (130 x 15) 1950 calories to maintain your weight.

You can use a food calorie chart to figure out the amount of calories contained in the food you eat. As we mentioned earlier, there are not only books and charts available that contain this information, but also a computer-analyzed **Nutrition Profile** from American Health and Nutrition.

For those interested in losing weight, this seven day food intake evaluation along with the **Exercise/Activity Evaluation**, encompass a Weight Control Program that can help you determine how many calories you should eat per day to get to your ideal weight, based on the personal information you provide.

DON'T COUNT CALORIES; MAKE CALORIES COUNT

When it comes to losing weight, too many people are too preoccupied with calories. Paul Stitt, biochemist and author of **Why Calories Don't Count**, states the problems behind the calorie-counting approach:

"Counting calories **won't** help you control your weight. That's because the organ in your body that controls hunger is blind to calories. Instead, it counts nutrients. Only when your body has enough of the 51 nutrients it needs will you feel full and satisfied.

Most calorie-counting dieters, however, usually eat low-nutrient, processed "diet" foods, so they never feel full. Instead, their skimpy meals leave them feeling hungry, weak and irritable. No wonder they can't stay on their diets.

That's why the best way to diet is to forget about calories. Instead, eat high-nutrient, high-fiber foods, such as fresh fruits and vegetables and whole grain breads...foods that satisfy you fast! That way you can eat until you're full and content, and still keep your calorie intake to a minimum."

You'll lose weight fast, and keep it off!

In the past, many people were told that if they avoided carbohydrates they would be able to maintain weight. Unfortunately, this is not true. Carbohydrates are some of the most nutritious foods we can eat. It is the refined carbohydrates that we need to avoid. Complex carbohydrates (fruits, vegetables, grains, nuts, seeds and beans) are low in calories and high in all nutrients, including protein, if you eat an adequate variety—all this without the fat. Diets high in fat can lead to many diseases.

ALL CALORIES ARE NOT CREATED EQUAL

The calories that complex carbohydrates contain are the most efficient fuel for energy and muscle building. Calories from sugars and fats have a tendency to build fat cells more than do those from complex carbohydrates.

Many people, perhaps due to a lack of vigorous exercise, poor diet, poor circulation, underactive glands or even inherited genetic problems do not burn calories at the same rate as others do. Their metabolism may be slower. These people will have to take in less calories than the standard charts show for their age and weight. This does not mean they will necessarily **always** burn calories slower, but until their bodies function at an optimal rate they will need to eat less calories.

Very often, individuals who had been slow metabolizers find that once they get their weight down to a normal ideal, their metabolism becomes more efficient and they will burn calories faster, allowing the individual to eat more calories without gaining extra weight. All of this must come from getting adequate exercise and eating the right foods, with emphasis on complex carbohydrates.

Another benefit of complex carbohydrates for weight control results from the fiber in these foods. Fiber helps the food residues to move through your intestines more efficiently, thus preventing some of the calories from being absorbed into your bloodstream.

Following is a sample comparison of foods high in nutrition versus those foods much lower in nutrition. Both categories of foods have approximately the same calorie count, (about 2400). This is the calorie requirement for an average American man who does an average amount of exercise or work. The average calorie intake for women is 1600. These are the calorie intake levels needed to maintain weight at present levels assuming a person is near his or her optimum weight. If you are above that weight, you must cut your calorie intake to at least the above figures or get more physical exercise, or a combination of both.

As you can see below, if you eat foods with less fats, sugars and unrefined flour, pasta and rice products, you will be able to eat **more** good healthy food than if you chose the lower nutrition meals with their extra high calorie counts. This is because your body metabolism is much more efficient when poor food choices are minimized. Fat intake of a typical meal can reduce oxygen availability by 25%. Not only is your metabolism and digestion slowed, but your physical endurance may be 3 times less than with a low fat diet.

Typical Breakfast-Approximately 700 Calories

High Nutrition Breakfast
1. One half grapefruit or 1 apple(eat 15 min. to ½ hour before meals for better digestion)
2. 2 eggs-softcooked preferred (light oil)
3. 2 oz. ham, or 2 oz. hard cheese, or small bowl oatmeal or other cooked whole grain flakes with ½ cup of milk and small amount of honey
4. 1 slice whole grain bread and 1 sq. of butter
5. 1 glass of 2% milk or ¼ cup plain lowfat yogurt

Lower Nutrition Breakfast
1. 3 hot cakes with butter and syrup
2. 1 cup coffee with ½ tsp. sugar and 2 tsp. cream, or 2 slices of bacon

Typical Lunch-Approximately 700 Calories

High Nutrition Lunch
1. 1 bowl of vegetable/lentil soup (just slightly cook vegetables)
2. 1 slice of whole grain bread with 1 sq. butter
3. ¼ cup of raw mixed nuts (soaked in water)
4. 1 cup of raw vegetables-chopped up in salad or whole with small amount of dressing. (carrots, celery, cauliflower, broccoli, etc., even potato)
5. ½ cup of plain yogurt or 2 oz. hard cheese

Lower Nutrition Lunch
1. 1 ham sandwich or small hamburger with bun and catsup
2. 1 soft drink or beer
3. 1 serving pie, cake, ice cream, etc.
4. 1 serving of french fries or hash browns fried in oil

Typical Dinner-Approximately 950 Calories

High Nutrition Dinner
1. 4 oz. tomato juice or 1 tomato
2. Mixed green salad with light herbal vinegar dressing. (ex. romaine lettuce, broccoli, parsley, spinach, watercress, greens, alfalfa sprouts)
3. 1 baked potato with butter. (Do not cook potato to dryness)
4. 5 oz. of lean roast beef or steak, or 8 oz. of seafood, or 6 oz. of baked tofu and 4 oz. of nut butter or tahini
5. 1 oz. cheddar or other hard cheese
6. 1 baked apple with ¼ cup whole milk

Lower Nutrition Dinner
1. Average serving of spaghetti and meatballs or 2 pieces of meatloaf
2. Mixed green salad with french dressing
3. Regular non-whole grain bread or French bread with butter
4. Small piece of cake, pie, whip'n chill, jello or ice cream
5. Coffee with cream or ½ glass of whole milk

The above meals under the "High Nutrition" heading are several times higher in protein and fiber, and are also higher in many of the vitamins and minerals.

There are books and charts available which have good tables for looking up the nutrient content of foods. American Health and Nutrition has developed a computer-analyzed **Nutrition Profile** (food intake evaluation) that evaluates your food consumption for the total amount of protein, complex carbohydrates, refined carbohydrates, dietary fat and fiber, and calorie intake over a one-week period. Along with the **Exercise/Activity Evaluation** which analyzes your calorie expenditure, you will have the information you need to lose, gain, or maintain your desired weight.

CALORIE MEASUREMENTS FOR WEIGHT LOSS

3,500 calories is equivalent to one pound of body fat. That is, when you burn 3,500 calories and don't take in any calories, you lose one pound of weight (excluding water loss). To say this another way, if you were to eat 500 less calories per day for seven days, you would lose one pound of weight per week; 1,000 less calories per day would result in two pounds of weight loss per week. This 500 calorie reduction could come from one or two less beers or one piece of pie (250 calories) and by adding a 45 minute brisk walk which can help you use up 250 calories. A one to two pound weight loss per week should be the maximum you aim for to be on the safe side.

HOW TO LOSE WEIGHT AND KEEP IT OFF

Almost half of all Americans are overweight. Some of us do not get enough exercise, some of us overeat, and others just eat the wrong foods. Overweight people show increased risk of death. Hypertension is the most potent risk factor for coronary heart disease, and it develops 10 times more often in persons who are 20% or more over their ideal weight.

If you follow all of the principles of good health as explained in this book, you will gradually and automatically reach your optimum weight - that weight which is best for your body. Some people even lose more weight than they think they should after changing their eating and living habits. But that is only because they're not used to seeing themselves slim. Your body will balance itself at whatever weight is best for your health, and you will not be deficient in nutrients.

Many people can lose weight temporarily by following the latest diet on the market or by not eating much for a period of time. These methods can deplete your body of nutrients needed for health and energy, and before long the weight will be back on again.

But taking off weight need not be a temporary thing. Nor does it have to be a particularly difficult thing to do, if you take the right approach. It has to become a way of life - sensible eating and exercising habits that eventually become second nature to you. If you're willing to face up to some simple but basic facts, you can cut through the nonsense and get at simple principles which can virtually assure that you will lose excess weight safely, and keep it off.

There are many diet or weight-loss centers around the country that can help if you'd like advice or would like to follow a specific program, but always look for one of these businesses that approaches weight-loss from a long term view of changing eating habits to eliminate extra weight causing foods, along with advice on proper exercise habits.

Eating what you like is a very satisfying pleasure, but eating what is healthy for you and that which has satisfying taste, is more than just pleasure. It gives you good health, happiness, and a longer, more energetic life.

To get extra pounds off and keep them off forever, there are several things you can do. Your diet has to stay low in fats, sugars, alcohol, and nutritionless foods that are high in calories. You should eat at the proper times and in the right amounts, and you must exercise often. When eating three or four smaller meals, your body will be able to metabolize and utilize the foods much more efficiently than when eating two large meals. The larger the meal the easier you put on fat.

Principles of Successful Weight Control

Give yourself time to think about how to get started on a weight reduction program and about all the benefits you will get. Become aware of the health problems that can result from being overweight - diabetes, high blood pressure, hardening of the arteries, poor circulation, thyroid problems, menstrual irregularities, low back pain, gallstones, breathing difficulties, etc. Think about how you became overweight and you'll be able to determine an appropriate approach. **Following are some points to help you:**

(1) Make a commitment to achieve your weight goal, have confidence in yourself, and have patience to wait for results.

(2) Be honest about how being overweight is really affecting your life-your physical appearance, your mood, your outlook on life, etc. Obesity is burdensome. It is damaging to health, drains you of pep and makes the average person feel, act and think older. You only have one chance to make a good 'first' impression. Recent studies show that others think that people who are healthy and slim are smarter and more likable. Your first impression is important in social life, personal relationships, and in business.

(3) Love yourself - you have to 'want' to look and feel better.

(4) Since weight control can take a lot of discipline, be sure to enjoy plenty of pleasurable 'nonfood' activities that will help you feel good about yourself.

(5) Visualize yourself being slim, and fitting into clothes you want to wear.

(6) Eat only what you want to eat. Don't eat to please others, whether it be the cook of the house, a hostess, or a waiter.

(7) Become aware of weaknesses in your eating habits that can lead to overeating.

(8) Strengthen your will power by gradually passing up small temptations like that extra spoonful of salad dressing or that piece of dessert.

(9) Learn new ways to shop and eat. The more you learn about food and nutrition, the easier it is to adopt better shopping and eating habits. And never shop when you're hungry.

(10) Save calories by substituting a low calorie food for high calorie food - for example, broiled fish instead of fried.

(11) Engage in some other activity when you get the urge to eat something you shouldn't. Occupy yourself with a hobby or chore, take a walk, or even go to the library.

(12) Leave the dishes of food in the kitchen. Take only your plate with food to the table.

(13) Keep high calorie and other junk foods out of reach and out of sight.

(14) Exercise everyday in your home or whereever you may be. Plan your day so you can make it a habit to exercise at least ten minutes to thirty minutes twice a day. Take as much time as you feel comfortable with and gradually you can increase it. Do not push exercise to an extreme however, in hopes of losing weight more quickly. But remember, exercise does burn off calories.

(15) Keep a positive attitude and praise yourself when you can see and feel your progress.

(16) Take a good health supplement to ensure your body of optimum levels of vitamins and minerals that you may not be getting when on a reduced calorie intake. A sufficient nutrient supply will keep your energy levels up and your body operating more effectively and efficiently.

(17) Don't take diet pills. The side effects can be uncomfortable and harmful, and they do not change your eating patterns, which is important for keeping weight off, once you've lost it.

(18) Drink water between meals to satisfy any hunger pangs.

(19) Consider having your total food consumption evaluated. This will tell you more about the total percentage of carbohydrates, fats and protein in your diet, your vitamin and mineral needs, and other nutritional factors, ranging from fiber to essential fatty acids. (You can write to American Health and Nutrition for information on a computerized food intake evaluation that will help you to determine your nutrient intake.)

Helpful Table Habits to Maintain Your Weight

If you enjoy eating, some of these suggestions can make that enjoyment last longer on less food.

(1) Taking your time and relaxing while eating.

(2) Savoring and chewing your food 30 to 50 times if you can. (This also helps digestion)

(3) Setting your fork or spoon down between bites.

(4) Taking a deep breath before each bite.

(5) Taking only small portions of calorie-rich foods, especially desserts and high fat foods.

(6) Not taking a second helping of anything.

(7) Eating small pieces of carrots, apples, or other fruits and vegetables for snacks.

By stretching your eating time, your stomach will have a chance to tell your brain that it's full, since it takes 20 minutes or so for your brain to react to this.

By concentrating on eating vegetables with abundant fiber, you can eat almost to your heart's content and not get too many calories. From there it depends on how much salad dressing, gravy or sauces that you put on your food. Try to get by with just a touch of this or a touch of that, or nothing at all.

Benefits of Fiber in Weight Control

Foods without fiber stay in your intestines longer, causing more calories to be absorbed. Foods rich in fiber will fill you up sooner.

There are two reasons for this. High fiber foods tend to require more chewing, so your eating time is slowed and your brain is given a chance to tell your body that you have had enough before you actually have eaten too much food. This fact is very important in weight control. High fiber foods also absorb and hold water while being digested. They tend to swell to a greater bulk than other foods and thus create a feeling of fullness that satisfies the appetite quicker with fewer calories. Fiber foods also stay in the stomach longer, thus helping to control the appetite.

Cooking Methods

Cooking methods also count in weight control and proper nutrition. Whenever possible, broil, bake or steam your foods rather than frying. Be careful not to dry out foods when cooking. For example, when you bake potatoes you can wrap them in foil to hold the moisture in. By retaining the moisture you will not have to use as much butter or other topping.

You can learn to enjoy foods without being fried. Fried foods are loaded with fats and oils from the frying process. If you do fry anything, use only a small amount of oil. All meats should have the fat trimmed off before cooking. You can enhance the flavor of foods cooked without fat by adding herbs or other seasonings.

Limit Fat and Sugar Intake

Other things you can do to avoid too much fat, saturated fat and cholesterol, are to choose lean meats and poultry, or more preferably, fish, skim milk, low fat yogurt and low fat cheese, dry beans, peas and nuts as your protein sources, along with eggs in moderation.

Also you should limit your use of butter, margarine, cream, shortening and foods made from such products. Read labels carefully to determine both amount and types of fat contained in foods. One way to cut down on butter is to blend one-fourth part vegetable oil with three-fourths part butter (cold processed, unrefined oil preferred).

Excess sugar intake is also detrimental to staying slim. Any sugar that you take in that is not used for energy as glucose turns into fat. Consequently you must limit your intake of sugar from all sources the way you must with fats, in order to reach and maintain correct weight.

In Summary

Exercise is also one of the most important factors in the ability to lose weight. The more aerobic exercise you do the more calories used and the more stored fat you burn up as energy.

One rule of thumb in losing weight is definite. **You must take in less calories than you burn.** No one should expect to, nor try to, lose weight too rapidly. You can develop many health problems from this type of behavior and you will be likely to regain weight.

Long term success depends on acquiring new and better habits of eating, drinking and exercise. Not only will you lose weight and become slender, but you will avoid a large number of health problems that result from being overweight as well.

Good luck!

BE SELECTIVE WHEN DINING OUT

When you dine at a restaurant, you must use discretion, not only in selecting your foods, but even in **choosing** the restaurant.

Reduce Fat and Salt

When selecting your foods, try to order those foods that are low in fats and oils and have had either little or no salt added. Try to stay away from foods with thick sauces. Select vegetables that are either raw or lightly cooked. Order soups that do not have meat stock as their base. These are high in fats and salt. Broiled and baked meats and fish are far more healthy than fried since they do not have the high fat content from the frying process. "Frying oils" used in many restaurants are usually used many times (up to 60) before being discarded. This makes the oil totally worthless for your health. It can and usually does become dirty, rancid and dangerous. Many restaurants even use oils made from petroleum by-products.

More Ideas To Help You Watch Your Weight

- Choose a drink such as sparkling water with a lemon twist instead of a cocktail. You don't need the calories, and since liquor tends to deaden the inhibitions, you may eat more than you intended too.
- Try to order first, so you won't be influenced by the choices of others in the party. Tune out their orders and don't change or add to your own.

- Order a la carte to get only the foods you want.
- Try selecting two or even three low-calorie appetizers instead of a full meal.
- Think twice before ordering highly spiced foods; they force you to drink too much, or to eat a sweet, in order to wash away the spicy taste.
- Choose foods that require you to work before you eat, such as unfilleted fish, crab legs in the shell, crayfish.
- If you're served large portions, eat only half of everything and ask the waiter to immediately put the portion you won't eat into a bag to be taken home and enjoyed at another meal.

Other Healthful Tips On Dining Out

Always ask for whole grain bread when possible, the house dressing (assuming it's made at the restaurant), and real milk for your coffee. Even the house dressing, or any dressing or sauce, should be used as lightly as possible. As for coffee, if you can get by without it, try to do so or drink only a small amount. If tempted by desserts, try sharing one between several people. You can do this at home too.

Never be afraid to ask for your food prepared the way you want it. You should always try to get the healthiest meals possible. After all, **you're** paying for them.

Many towns and cities have natural food restaurants where the food is very nutritious and is prepared with proper care. Always try to go to a restaurant where those concerns are not taken lightly.

TYPICAL NUTRIENT-BALANCED DIET

The easy way to be sure one is getting a good diet is by following a food guide. The following guide groups together foods of similar nutrient content and shows how many servings of each group should be chosen each day for necessary nutrients. Single meals or whole daily menus may be planned using this guide.

Including a variety of choices from the following food groups in your daily diet helps to insure a balanced nutrient intake.

1. Beans, nuts, seeds, eggs, meats (including fish and poultry)
   One serving is any of the following:

- ½ cup cooked dry beans, lentils, or tofu
- ½ cup nuts or seeds
- ½ cup tuna or 4 oz. seafood

- 2 eggs
- 4 tbsp. peanut butter
- 4 oz. lean meat or poultry

Calorie range: 140 for 2 eggs to 400 for peanut butter   **2 or 3 servings**

2. Tofu or dairy products (especially cultured foods — yogurt, cheese, etc.)
One serving is:
- 1 cup tofu, yogurt or milk
- 1½ oz. of cheddar cheese

Calorie range: 75 for tofu to 165 for cheddar cheese   **2 servings**

3. Whole grains and cereals
One serving is:
- 1 slice whole grain bread
- ½ cup cooked cereal
- ½ cup cooked brown rice
  or whole grain macaroni (pasta)
- 4 crackers or 1 pancake or 1 roll
- ¾ cup dry cereal

Calorie value: 70   **4 to 6 servings**

4. High-starch vegetables
One serving is:
- ½ cup corn, potato, beets, carrots, yams, peas, squash or green beans

Calorie value: 70   **1 or 2 servings**

5. Other vegetables (especially dark green)
One serving is:
- 1 cup broccoli, cabbage, greens, brussel sprouts, asparagus
- 1½ to 2 cups romaine lettuce or spinach
- 2 tomatoes
- ½ cup green pepper

Calorie value: 40   **2 servings**

6. Fruits
One serving is:
- 1 apple, peach, pear, banana, orange or 4 prunes

Calorie value: 40   **2 servings**

7. Fats and oils
One serving is:
- 1 tbsp. vegetable oil, butter or mayonnaise

Calorie value: 100   **1 serving**

Note: Many foods are not included here. The foods listed are only examples. This guide provides between 1100 and 2000 calories per day, depending on the choices within food groups. Persons who need more calories should choose more or larger servings. Persons who need fewer calories should consider increasing their activity level, rather than reducing their food intake.

See the back of this book for an extensive food chart showing calories, protein and fat content of some common foods.

Experiment with calorie levels until you find an optimum amount to consume to get to and stay at your ideal weight. Weigh yourself once each week to see how you're doing.

There are many excellent recipe cookbooks on the market to help you prepare super nutritious and healthful meals. You'll find the largest selection of these in health food stores. Some of our recommendations are **Recipes For A Small Planet, Deaf Smith**

Country Cookbook, and **Laurel's Kitchen.** Our favorite and our top recommendation is **FOR THE LOVE OF FOOD** by Jeanne Martin. You can write to us for a free description of these and other books on healthful living.

SMOKING

Everyone knows smoking is dangerous and "hazardous to your health". However, smoking is more than just hazardous to your health — it can kill you long before your time. Sure, there are individuals who say "I've smoked tobacco all my life, and I'm healthy", but it is only rare that smokers will not find their bodies gradually deteriorating. Not only will their lungs become ulcerated but the immune system and organs in their bodies will deteriorate from the by-products of smoke and from the hundreds of toxic poisons inherent in tobacco. Lead, cadmium and aluminum are highly toxic metals emitted in tobacco smoke. This alone is reason enough to not even breathe secondary smoke. Pipe tobacco and cigars cause most of the same health problems. Even the mouth and throat can become cancerous from the heat, smoke and toxins in tobacco. Smoking marijuana is likely to be as bad for your mouth, throat, and especially lungs as tobacco is.

Following are some additional consequences of smoking:

(1) Emphysema from the effects of smoking will eventually leave you out of breath and exhausted. Eventually, a heavy smoker can suffocate due to the lack of lung capacity.

(2) Miscarriages are twice as common when mothers smoke heavily. Lower birth weights and increased birth defects can also occur.

(3) Smokers have a two to three times greater chance of dying from a heart attack.

(4) Smokers have twenty-five times the chance of developing lung cancer as non-smokers.

(5) The death rate for smokers taking birth control pills is about six times that for nonsmokers.

(6) Female smokers experience menopause at much younger ages.

(7) Smokers lose some of their sense of taste and smell, and develop more facial wrinkles.

(8) There is an increased risk of contracting viruses, germs, etc. due to a greatly reduced immune system response.

Studies have shown that smoking does not calm nerves and does not improve mood or performance.

Some people think smoking helps them function at higher mental levels. But smoking only allows the smoker to reach the level of mental functioning comparable to that of a nonsmoker. It only has a calming effect in the sense that it relieves some of the agitation and irritation associated with withdrawal.

To stop smoking, you must want to stop and have confidence in your ability to stop. Smoking injures and kills. If you love life, you'll do all you can to rid yourself of this very dangerous habit.

CARE OF YOUR TEETH AND MOUTH

The most important thing to keep in mind about dental care is to eat nutritious foods that have plenty of minerals and to avoid foods with high amounts of sugars. If you do eat sugary foods, be sure to rinse your mouth well afterwards and brush if you can, even if it is only with water. This same routine should ideally apply to any foods you eat, although the sugary foods create bacteria more quickly. Some foods have actually been found to inhibit bacteria, particularly some cheeses and nuts. However, that doesn't mean you should leave cheddar cheese residue in your mouth.

The reason we mention eating foods high in minerals, or perhaps even supplementing your diet with moderate amounts of minerals, is that a number of minerals are needed for strong healthy teeth and enamel, and better decay resistance. Regular tooth brushing means brushing at least once a day, and more if you have the oportunity. A side benefit of regular tooth brushing (and flossing) is a fresher breath.

To brush correctly, place the bristles at a 45 degree angle with your gums and place into the gum line. Massage gently back and forth to extract food residue and bacteria, then brush upward or downward **with** the teeth. A medium soft tooth brush is best. Be sure to brush your tongue everyday as well - another aid to a clean mouth!

Flossing should be done at least every couple of days but preferably on a daily basis. Flossing gets the bacteria and food residue out from between the teeth and on the teeth down to the gum lines. Floss gently so you do not damage your gums. Unwaxed floss is best. Extra Vitamin C in your diet can also help to prevent gum disease and resultant tooth decay. Lastly—visit a dentist regularly.

SKIN AND BODY CARE

The normal and healthy self-image that begins to form when we first realize what a mirror is, stays with us through the years as we all try to be like the person we know is within us. Consequently, it is just human nature for us to spend our lives working to improve our appearance — at least we should try to.

Beauty, a good complexion, healthy looking skin and hair, and a clean smelling mouth all start from **within** the body, not from trying to use tons of products on the outside. Good nutrition and regular exercise are prerequisites to good looks.

Beauty (in both men and women) is a radiance and reflection of good health, and health comes from within.

Just as food with artificial colors, oils and other chemicals is not healthy for your "inner" body, chemicalized body care products are **also** damaging to your skin and hair. In fact, many people become ill or develop allergies from many commercial products on the market. Even some commercial mouthwashes were recently pointed out as causing cancerous lesions in the mouth.

The delicate environment of your skin, hair, and mouth exists best in its own natural state. So any products you use on or in them should be made up of natural ingredients. Some of these ingredients are aloe vera, jojoba, herbs, proteins, coconut, avocado, etc. Hand soaps made from natural glycerine, for instance, are preferable to damaging detergent soaps.

Health food stores were the first places that tried to provide these highest quality body care products. Most of them still carry the safest and most effective products available, although these types of products are now becoming available from a few other quality-conscious suppliers.

It is still very important to read the labels and ask what the ingredients are if you're not familiar with them. For instance, in skin moisturizers some of the best natural ingredients that help to make your skin look its youngest are elastin, collagen, placenta, and NaPCA, most of which you may not recognize. Sometimes you will find just a small amount of preservative in a product which might be necessary to keep it fresh longer. Other effective skin moisturizing ingredients might be aloe vera, jojoba, herbal oils, and vegetable oils. These ingredients actually feed your skin and hair from the outside with essential nutrients and keep your skin looking healthier and younger. Chemicalized products can do just the opposite and can leave your skin and hair dried out and unhealthy.

Natural ingredients are usually more costly than petroleum and chemical derived products, but most often you get what you pay for. Besides the usual products referred to above — shampoos, conditioners, lotions, etc. — other products that are now available with safe quality ingredients are natural toothpastes, eyewashes, mouthwashes, insect repellents, healing salves, and many, many other items.

Always remember that along with the use of quality body care products, good nutrition and regular exercise, you need to avoid five other causes of aging skin and lifeless hair — stress, alcohol, smoking, excess sun and rapid weight loss.
Here's to a good-looking you!

FOOD ALLERGIES

Earlier in the book we mentioned that some people are allergic to the gluten in wheat and some other grains. We also mentioned that some people are allergic to milk. That is, they cannot digest the lactose in milk. In both cases, they may have sensitivity reactions or symptoms when eating these foods.

More common foods that can cause minor to major allergic reactions are yeast, citrus, tomatoes, eggs, nuts, alcohol, protein, beef, chocolate, bananas and many others. Good eating habits such as eating slowly, chewing your food thoroughly, not overeating, and most of the others listed in the **Summary of Good Eating Habits** section will improve the digestion of these foods, and therefore minimize allergic reactions to them. A good digestive enzyme supplement can also be helpful in aiding your digestion.

Many people experience ill-health symptoms that may be related to food or chemical allergies but they don't know it. These can range from headaches and asthma to arthritis symptoms. Sometimes these symptoms do not show up for days or even years, until finally your body's cells can no longer handle the stress of the biochemical imbalances caused by the sensitivity to food. If you detect allergies early enough, you may be able to avoid any permanent damage to your body. It is very difficult to check for food allergies, but this can either be done through expensive blood and skin tests or through testing for them in your diet. You can do this yourself or you may want to do it under the guidance of your doctor.

Clinical ecologists have concluded that many food sensitivities result from eating a food too often. This is a very good reason to eat as varied a diet as possible and refrain from eating the same foods every day. Some foods may cause reactions no matter how seldom you eat them. You may be best off eliminating these from your diet entirely. For example, some artificial colors are common offenders for some people.

If you suspect a certain food, first eliminate it from your diet for a week or so. When you eat it again, you will be more sensitive to that food. If it causes symptoms, eliminate it for 90 days and try again. If no symptoms appear you will have become desensitized to that food and will then be able to include it in your diet on a limited basis. If you do have a reaction after 90 days it is best to eliminate it entirely. It can be very worthwhile to test for food allergies if you suspect you may have this problem, since these types of allergies can result in premature aging and degenerative diseases.

CHEMICAL ALLERGIES

As many as one-third of all allergies may be caused by chemicals in our home or work place. Avoid contact with chemicals in household products such as cleansers, soaps, paint, etc. Avoid breathing fumes and contact with skin. It is a good idea to store as many of these as possible outside your house in a garage or shed to avoid possible exposure, especially if you may be sensitive. A good nutritional supplement may also help to eliminate some toxins from the body, but avoiding toxins as much as possible is the best medicine.

Some cosmetics and body care products also contain ingredients that can cause reactions. Be sure to use those that contain only natural substances. Again it is a good idea to vary the products you use so as not to build a sensitivity to a particular ingredient. It is even a good idea to use non-colored and non-scented facial tissue and toilet paper to avoid the chemical scents and colors.

Following the methods we've mentioned, you should be able to minimize troublesome symptoms and lead a healthy life. By being aware of symptoms you may experience, you will be able to check each new food or other product that you introduce into your life.

NONTOXIC BIODEGRADABLE HOUSEHOLD PRODUCTS

Many commercial soaps, cleaners and germicides can be very toxic and irritating, and those that are relatively safe are nonbiodegradable and contain phosphates, meaning they do not break down when reaching the sewer systems before they are returned to the environment. Phosphate-containing products choke off plant and fish life.

There are a number of biodegradable, noncaustic and nontoxic products on the market which are even more effective at cleaning, deodorizing or whatever the application may be.

NONCHEMICALIZED GARDENING PRODUCTS

Just about everyone is aware of the dangers and toxicity of commercial farm and garden insecticides, herbicides, and pesticides. Many allergies can be attributed to chemicals in the environment. Gardening and farming can be done organically — that is, without the use of harmful ingredients.

Natural and organic gardening and farming also entails the use of crop rotation, vegetation residue from previous years, natural fertilizers such as manure, grass, leaves, garbage, mineral-bearing rock such as soft rock phosphate, seaweed, fish emulsion, natural plant hormones, soil enzymes, and biological pest control management.

If you would like more information on safe and effective gardening and farming products and methods or on nontoxic household products write to: American Health and Nutrition, 7 North Pinckney St., Suite 225, Madison, Wisconsin 53703.

ANTI-OXIDANTS CAN HELP PREVENT AGING

Chemical reactions are continually burning fuel in our bodies' cells and are controlled by certain enzyme systems that are also referred to as anti-oxidants. This means they slow down or control the rate at which oxygen is burned from the energy stored in the cells. The lower we keep that rate, the longer and healthier we will live.

Radiation from various sources, chemicals and other toxins that act to speed this oxidation of our cells can form damaging substances in our body called free radicals. They can form from pollutants, poisons, rancid oils, certain chemical reactions within our body, and even from foods we eat. The better our nutritional habits are the stronger our cells and cell membranes will be to withstand attack by free radicals. Many nutrients, especially vitamins A,C,E, the mineral Selenium, the enzymes Super-oxide Dismutase, (S.O.D.) and Catalase, and the amino acids Cysteine, Methionine and Glutathione help to neutralize free radicals. S.O.D. and Catalase are available in liquid form in order to be better assimilated by the body and to avoid destruction in the stomach.

Because of the increase of free radicals in our environment today, there is a need to counter their effects to help us stay younger longer.

PREVENT CANCER
THROUGH HEALTHFUL LIVING

We have already discussed many factors that have a possible part in causing cancer. Each year cancer, the most feared of all diseases, claims approximately 400,000 lives. Yet, it is one of the most easily preventable diseases. Research has indicated that many forms of cancer result from toxins and carcinogens in our food supply, the water we drink and the air we breathe. Many toxins and cancer-causing substances act as 'free radicals' in the body that have the ability to damage the genetic control system within the cell (DNA&RNA). This damage allows individual cells to reproduce as mutant cancerous cells. The healthier we can keep our cells with sufficient vitamins, minerals, oxygen and other nutrients, the easier they can withstand attack by carcinogens.

Studies on death due to cancer confirm the importance of lifestyle. Practicing Mormons and Seventh-Day Adventists do not smoke or drink alcohol or coffee. Their diet consists of plenty of grains, fruits and vegetables and very little meat. Apparently as a result of this lifestyle, they have a cancer rate of only 50 percent of that for the general population. The incidence of lung, colon, rectal, breast, ovarian and uterine cancers are all extremely low.

Effects Of Diet

The National Cancer Institute has found that "diet and nutrition appear to account for the largest number of human cancers." The National Academy of Sciences and the American Cancer Society have also issued reports, based on extensive research of thousands of studies by hundreds of scientists, that indicate a probable and possible relationship between the foods we eat and the incidence of cancer. Diet may be one of the most significant factors in avoiding and possibly reversing this disease.

T. Colin Campbell, a nutritional biochemist at the Cornell University Nutrition Institute and a member of the National Academy of Sciences, has stated that although environmental factors cause most people to form mutant cells in their bodies, their risk for developing cancer can be increased by as much as 10 times depending upon their diet. He has also reported that high consumption of fats and protein are believed to promote cancer, and that fruits and vegetables rich in vitamins A, C and E can prevent and may reverse growth of cancerous cells. He says a diet high in fiber from whole grain cereals, nuts, seeds, legumes, fruits and vegetables may inhibit certain cancers.

The National Academy of Sciences 'Diet and Cancer' report stated that studies have shown that vegetables in the cabbage family—cabbage, brussel sprouts, broccoli, cauliflower and kale—increase the body's output of cancer-inhibiting enzymes. They recommend that people should also eat more of these foods regularly.

Research has linked cancer of the stomach and esophagus in Japan and other countries to **excess salt** consumption. Too much of anything can have a destructive effect on our cells.

Many studies have shown a direct association between high-fat diets (saturated or unsaturated) and breast cancer, colon cancer and prostate cancer.

In countries where people consume large amounts of nitrite-cured or smoked foods, there is high incidence of cancer of the stomach or esophagus. These foods may contain certain chemicals, nitrosamines and hydrocarbons that are suspected of being carcinogenic (cancer-causing) in humans.

Molds on food are also potentially dangerous. Either cut **well beyond** mold spots on food or better yet, throw it away entirely. Another type of mold to be aware of is **aflatoxin.** It is most commonly found in peanuts. Though the federal government has set standards on maximum aflatoxin levels, small amounts of fungus may still be present. Our suggestion is to minimize your intake of peanuts or better yet, purchase peanuts from suppliers that try to provide peanuts with low aflatoxin levels. Arrowhead Mills (Deaf Smith) is one company we are familiar with, and because they sun-dry their peanuts, mold problems are avoided.

Fats

Some research studies have shown that smoke generated from fat dripping on hot charcoal coals can produce potentially carcinogenic chemicals that end up in the food you are grilling.

Rancidity or spoiling of foods containing oils and fats may also be the cause of the development of cancer cells in the gastric or stomach area. Since polyunsaturated fats oxidize, or turn rancid much sooner than saturated fats, high consumption of these fats are the ones most likely to cause certain types of cancer. Even skin cancer has been linked to rancidity of fat in body tissues. Heat and oxygen in the body, along with ultraviolet radiation from the sun, or other sources of radiation acclerate the oxidation of fats causing damage (mutation) to the tissues, thus stimulating cancer and aging of the skin. Anything that acts as an anti-oxidant will help prevent this damage from occurring. Vitamin E is a very good antioxidant that is found naturally in many whole foods with a high unsaturated fat content: nuts, grains, seeds, legumes, etc.

(Another section in this book discusses other nutrients involved with preventing oxidation.)

Heating polyunsaturated fats like corn or safflower, as in cooking, will immediately cause the oil to become rancid and damaging to the body. Though they do have other beneficial effects for your circulatory system, heart and blood vessels, as well as in moisturizing the body, it is not a good idea to fry with them. Frying with very low heat for a short period of time may be okay, but we suggest using monounsaturated oils such as sesame or olive oil (Olive oil is our recommendation). Always heat oils at the lowest temperature you can and never use more than what you need to. Of course, saturated fats are even better for heating, again as long as you watch how much you use so as not to overburden your body with saturated fats. Even these fatty acids break down when exposed to high heat as in deep-frying. We strongly suggest that you avoid deep-fat frying as much as possible, as well as any other fried foods.

'Live' Foods

Eating plenty of raw fruits and vegetables has been shown to decrease the incidence of stomach and other cancers by as much as 35 percent. Dr. Ann Wigmore of the Hippocrates Health Institute in Boston incorporates a diet of 'live', uncooked fruits, vegetables, fermented foods and sprouts of grains and seeds to nourish the body on the cellular level with the nutrients, enzymes and bacteria needed to increase the effectiveness of the immune system in fighting cancers, thus allowing the body to heal itself. The fiber in these foods also prevents colon cancer because the fiber sweeps the intestines clean of the toxins.

Charles Shaw M.D. of the University of Texas Cancer Center, found that cancer cells do not grow in the presence of chlorophyll, the green pigment found in green vegetables, sprouts and grasses such as wheat grass.

Poor nutrition, stress and lack of exercise can all play a part in weakening your immune system and allow toxins to develop that can eventually cause cancer.

There is much documentation in the medical literature in support of the effectiveness of raw thymus extract in promoting the health of the immune system. This extract is available in either liquid or tablet form, with the liquid being most effective. There is considerable research going on studying the possible benefits of glandular, organ, bone marrow and other tissue extracts in the treatment of corresponding cancers.

Coffee And Alcohol

What we drink is as important as what we eat. Excess **coffee** drinking has been linked to pancreatic cancer. **Alcohol** can produce liver cancer after cirrhosis of the liver has developed. It also increases the risk of cancer of the throat, mouth and esophagus. Even beer drinking has been shown to have a definite correlation with colon and rectal cancer. This could be from any number of elements: aritificial colorings, preservatives, nitrate formations or some element that has not yet been isolated.

Drinking or eating **foods that are too hot** can also damage cells in the mouth, throat, esophagus and stomach and may cause cancer to develop. As you can see, whenever cells are damaged, there is a possibility of cancer developing.

Smoking

For both men and women the risk of getting lung cancer is **directly** related to smoking. Smoking cigars, pipes and cigarettes, as well as **chewing** tobacco, increases the risk of mouth, throat, larynx, esophagus and bladder cancers.

Estrogen

Long term use of **estrogen** for menopause increases the risk of uterine cancer. By keeping your body in optimal health through all the suggestions we've given, you will be able to avoid or minimize the use of estrogen.

Drugs

Even some **prescription drugs** can initiate cancer through certain reactions in the body. For example, some ulcer drugs reduce acidity in the stomach thereby permitting growth in the stomach of bacteria that can form carcinogenic nitrosamines.

Radiation

There are over 400,000 new cases of skin cancer each year. The prime cause is excess ultraviolet radiation from sunlight. Most cases occur on those parts of the body most often exposed to the sun such as face, ears, back of hands and neck. Excess radiation from X-rays increases the risk of getting leukemia and thyroid cancer.

Chemicals And Pollution

The environment is becoming a major threat in causing cancer. As much as 50 percent of cancers may be environmentally related. Deaths due to lung cancer are several times more frequent in Los Angeles than Chicago, most likely do to the difference in air pollution. Pollutants and chemicals like DES, PCB, Dioxin, saccharin, nitrosamines, auto fumes, herbicides, pesticides, food additives, etc. have taken their toll. And the nightmare of industrial chemicals and wastes is a horror we're just now starting to realize the extent of. Exposure to industrial agents and chemicals are known to increase cancer risk for certain occupations. For example:

-People who work in rubber and aniline dye plants develop more bladder cancer.

-Woodworkers and nickel miners develop more sinus cancer.

-Uranium, asbestos workers and roofers develop more lung cancer.

-Vinyl chloride workers develop more liver cancer.

Nutritional Deficiencies

Besides cancers caused by the environment and by chemicals, there are many cancers that result from nutrient deficiencies. According to recent statistics from the U.S. Department of Health, Education and Welfare (HEW) and the U.S. Department of Agriculture, the following nutritional deficiencies have been found to increase the probability of cancer:

- Choline deficiency leads to higher incidence of liver cancer.
- Vitamin E deficiency causes leukemia cancer to increase.
- Iodine deficiency leads to increased cancer of the thyroid.
- A deficiency of the B-Vitamins can cause liver damage and malignancies.
- Zinc deficiency increases chances of prostate cancer.
- A deficiency of pro-Vitamin A has been linked to a higher incidence of lung cancer. Evidence continues to mount showing that fruits and vegetables rich in beta-carotene, (pro-Vitamin A), may help prevent lung cancer and other cancers. Best fruit and vegetable sources of pro-Vitamin A are listed in the Vitamin and Mineral Guide of this book.

- Statistical data gathered by the National Cancer Institute has indicated that Selenium deficiency in the diet may lead to several forms of cancer. This is due to selenium's function as a free radical scavenger (anti-oxidant) in protecting the body's cells.

Protect Yourself Against Cancer

Early detection is the key to increasing chances of cancer cures. The earlier a cancer is found, the greater chance for treatment to work. Detecting cancer early is not as difficult as it might seem.

Know The Seven Common Warning Signals of Cancer

(These symptoms do not necessarily indicate cancer.)
Change in bowel or bladder habits.
A sore that does not heal.
Unusual bleeding or discharge.
Thickening or lump in breast or elsewhere.
Indigestion, difficulty in swallowing.
Obvious change in wart or mole.
Nagging cough or hoarseness.
Many cancers have specific symptoms other than these seven common ones. If you have any unusual symptoms that persist for even two weeks, we suggest you see your doctor.

Even if you have no symptoms, it would be wise to have cancer-related checkups. The American Cancer Society suggests a checkup every three years for people between the ages of 20 and 40 and every year for those 40 and over.

You Can Help Yourself Prevent Cancer

Eating for good health and prevention of cancer may take a bit more imagination and thought on the part of the cook, but if it lowers your family's risk of cancer, the challenge is well worth it.

Your local American Cancer Society and the Cancer Control Society of 2043 North Berendo Street, Los Angeles, CA 90027 will provide helpful information to you on preventing, controlling and coping with cancer.

If we can change or eliminate any of the many risk factors, we can reduce the incidence of cancer. Because there are so many factors that can be involved, prevention as well as treatment should encompass many approaches including stress reduction, improved diet, etc. not just cancer checkups, chemotherapy and other medical treatments. Without removing the **cause** of the cancer (toxins, stress, malnourishment of the cells, destructive lifestyle habits, environmental pollutants), medical treatment will not help. There is a place for surgery, radiation and chemotherapy, but they have all been over emphasized at the expense of natural alternatives.

Modern medicine should combine all therapies for a more holistic approach that will help to **build** the immune system rather than to destroy it. Whatever we can do to improve the health and purity of our bloodstream will improve the health of our cells to enable them to ward off carcinogens. The most effective treatment for any disease is accomplished by our own body's extensive healing mechanism. Your job is to provide the proper conditions necessary to support, stimulate and activate the body's own healing activity.

Be sure you don't get the feeling that "since just about everything causes cancer, it's useless to try to avoid it". Having a strong, positive mental attitude is very important in preventing and treating cancer. By visualizing cancer cells as weak and yourself as being strong, you can actually trigger chemical reactions in your body that can aid in preventing and fighting cancer cells. Of course, other 'proper' conditions must also be incorporated into your life. If we would all act and live our lives as though there were already cancer cells growing in our bodies, we would then be doing everything necessary to prevent cancer from actually occurring in the first place.

THE IMPORTANCE OF HEALTH SUPPLEMENTS

Many people don't know why vitamins and minerals are essential for life. Once you understand the importance of vitamins and minerals, you will be more concerned about getting enough of them. A multiple vitamin-mineral supplement will help to prevent minor symptoms, disease and even stress-related problems. Doctors agree that the body will make use of additional vitamins during times of need, if they are available.

Government and independent studies show that even without a *classical* vitamin deficiency disease, an individual may suffer from a **marginal** or latent, **vitamin deficiency.**

This condition, which has only been identified in recent years, may affect the body's ability to resist disease and infection, to recover from surgery, stress or disease, or to engage in high-level thinking.

This marginal state of vitamin depletion sometimes is not obvious, because it causes only vague symptoms such as lethargy, irritability, insomnia and difficulty in concentrating. You can look healthy, but be on the way to serious illness. The *Journal of the American Medical Association* pointed out recently that the deficiency of a single vitamin has a profound effect in decreasing the response of the immune system, thus making us more likely to get infections from viruses and bacteria and perhaps become more susceptible to cancer.

Physical and emotional stress, medications, pollution, eating junk food (refined sugar and flour products, fried foods, etc.) and overcooking your food all rob your body of essential nutrient supplies. Many nutrients actually draw pollutant chemicals and toxic metals like lead, mercury and cadmium out of the body. Some of these are vitamins A, C and E, Selenium, Methionine and Cysteine. Fiber, fruit pectin and algin from sea vegetables like kelp, also help to absorb toxic metals. Very few people lead such a perfectly healthy lifestyle or live in such clean environments that they would not benefit from vitamin supplementation.

Some would argue that if we eat enough of the right foods, all of our vitamins are supplied. As Earl Mindell, pharmacist, nutritionist and author of the *Vitamin Bible* and *Vitamin Bible For Your Kids* says, "We simply aren't able to eat as much of the vitamin-rich foods necessary to supply all of our needs. It is foolish to believe that the foods found on the supermarket shelves can supply all of these elements essential to life itself."

The USDA Nationwide Food Consumption Survey of 1979 supports the contention that the average American isn't even meeting the Recommended Daily Allowance for many nutrients through dietary sources.

Why Take Vitamin Supplements

Thorough evaluation of the medical and scientific literature suggests that for most vitamins and minerals, current RDA levels are inadequate to be effective in reducing the incidence of many other diseases, including the two most serious nutrition-related illnesses — cardiovascular diseases and many types of cancer.

It is the personal responsibility of everyone of us to maintain our own health. Vitamin supplementation is our nutritional insurance to help balance your unique body chemistry. You can help your body to resist disease, illness and infection and recover from ailments more rapidly with an adequate supply of nutrients.

In his book, SUPERNUTRITION, nationally-respected biochemist and nutritionist Dr. Richard Passwater states that "500,000 to 1,000,000 lives could be saved each year if we supplemented our diets above the minimum RDA". He says "most individuals would live better lives, live longer lives, stay younger longer and be happier."

The research and clinical experience of many doctors, nutritionists and biochemists have shown that groups of people who supplement their diet with vitamins and minerals to help balance body chemistry are generally healthier than those who try to get enough from food alone. Most of these people are stronger, more intelligent, healthier looking, more resistant to sickness and disease, and even better problem solvers than other groups not supplementing their diet.

Research has also shown that as people grow older, their systems often fail to use those nutrients available in their foods to best advantage. Consequently, they require either a greater quantity of food or supplementation of nutrients, especially Vitamin C, calcium, Vitamin D, iron, zinc, folic acid and vitamin B-12.

Summary of Reasons for Supplementation:
1. Poor digestion and poor absorption of nutrients.
2. Refining and processing of foods.
3. Improper cooking methods — boiling, frying, reheating and overcooking.
4. Imbalances — excess of some nutrients, lack of others.
5. Interferences with utilization - pesticides, alcohol, smoking, drugs, oral contraceptives.
6. Harvesting unripe fruits and vegetables.
7. Improper storage of foods.
8. Lack of variety in the diet.
9. Depletion of nutrients due to physical and mental stress.
10. Soil nutrient depletion due to poor agricultural practices.
11. Excess sugar intake.
12. Biochemical individuality.
13. Prevention of marginal nutrient deficiencies.
14. Elimination of toxic metals and chemicals.
15. To strengthen the immune system (resist disease and infection.
16. Recovery from surgery, stress, illness and physical exertion.
17. To help you think more clearly and control mood swings.
18. Reduced food and nutrient intake when dieting.
19. To help protect the body's cells from oxidation (aging).

As we can see, it takes much larger amounts of vitamins and minerals than the minimum RDAs to counter all the factors listed above. People who think we only need a small amount of nutrients are behind the times in their knowledge of the role of vitamins and minerals, and forget to take these factors into account.

Suggestions For Health Supplements

We feel that everyone could benefit from a basic program of supplementation as a foundation for insuring a sufficient amount of vitamins, minerals, digestive enzymes, and glandular and organ support for their bodies, even though they may have no obvious deficiencies or symptoms.

The suggested amounts of nutrients listed below can be obtained through food sources, supplementation, or best of all, a combination of both.

Following is a range of dosages usually available in various formulas, that we feel may be appropriate in promoting super-health:

VITAMINS	DOSAGE	MINERALS	DOSAGE
Vitamin A	10,000-25,000 I.U.	Calcium	300-1000 mg.
Vitamin D	400-1,000 I.U.	Phosphorous	75-150 mg.
Vitamin C	500-3,000 mg.	Magnesium	170-500 mg.
Vitamin E	50-400 I.U.	Potassium	99 mg.
B Complex		Iron	15-30 mg.
Vitamin B-1	25-50 mg.	Iodine	.15-.225 mg.
Vitamin B-2	25-100 mg.	Copper	.5-2 mg.
Vitamin B-6	25-100 mg.	Manganese	10-20 mg.
Vitamin B-12	25-100 mcg.	Zinc	15-25 mg.
Niacin or	25-100 mg.	Chromium	50-200 mcg.
Niacinamide (B-3)		Selenium	50-200 mcg.
Pantothenic Acid	25-100 mg.	**Other Nutrients**	
Folic Acid	400 mcg.	Betaine	15-150 mg.
Biotin	100-300 mcg.	Hydrochloride	
Choline	25-100 mg.	Bioflavonoids	50-500 mg.
Inositol	25-100 mg.		
Paba	25-100 mg.		

Glandular and Organ Supplements

Ovarian (for women)	60 mg.	Heart	60 mg.
Prostate (for men)	60 mg.	Lungs	60 mg.
Thymus	60 mg.	Kidney	60 mg.
Pancreas	60 mg.	Liver	60 mg.
Adrenal	60 mg.	Brain	60 mg.
Pituitary	10 mg.	Spleen	60 mg.
Thyroid	100 mg.		

Digestion Aids

Betaine	60-325 mg.	Bile	65 mg.
Hydrochloride		Rennin	15 mg.
Pancreatin	75 mg.	Mycozyme	35 mg.
Pepsin	35-135 mg.	Lipase	50 mg.
Papain	50 mg.		

We feel that a multiple supplement has many advantages over a combination of individual supplements. You will know that you are getting all the nutrients at the same time for maximum effectiveness, and you will have fewer bottles to keep track of.

It is also more economical than taking all the nutrients individually.

The *multivitamin and mineral supplement* is intended to accommodate a wide variation in nutritional requirements by providing a *full complement* of the essential vitamins and minerals. Taken daily, a properly formulated multivitamin and mineral supplement will give the body an opportunity to absorb everything it requires in the way of micronutrients and eliminate what it does not need.

We suggest that you do not take individual nutrients in very high dosages without first consulting a nutrition consultant, nutritionist or other health care professional, or unless it has been recommended to you through a reputable nutritional evaluation.

If you want to start on a vitamin program, we suggest that you begin with a high quality vitamin-mineral supplement with moderate potencies. You can add individual supplements such as Vitamin C and E and others and gradually increase the dosage you are taking until you feel you have reached what is best for you.

If you are following a program of total health and a supplementation program, it's still possible that you may have particular symptoms of ill-health. A nutritional evaluation based on body signs and symptoms would be useful to identify a particular nutrient deficiency. You could then increase your intake of that nutrient until your symptoms have subsided. For more information on this kind of evaluation, please see the section in this book that explains computerized health appraisals.

You must decide for yourself at which level of nutritional supplementation you feel and function best. Following good nutritional guidelines and leading a healthy lifestyle will help you lower the amount of supplementation you may need.

Proper Use of Health Supplements

Generally, most supplements should be taken with your meals. This is important for several reasons. There are usually nutrients in many foods that synergistically aid in the absorption of vitamins and minerals. Some of the better supplements have small amounts of different foods, herbs, etc. added to them for this reason. As we've said, you need fats and oils to aid in the assimilation of Vitamins A, D, E and K. By taking the supplements with your meals you will also avoid the slightly queasy stomach that some people experience when taking them on an empty stomach.

Hydrochloric acid is secreted by the stomach to aid in the digestion of your meal. This is important because an acid environment in the stomach is necessary for absorbing the calcium that is part of the supplement.

Taking all the vitamins and minerals in a balanced tablet or capsule is the best method of supplementation. Taking a multivitamin at least twice per day with meals is better than taking a supplement once a day. This will provide nutrients to your body more evenly so they will be better utilized and assimilated.

Sustained-release supplements are available and are designed to disintegrate gradually in the digestive tract. However, even a sustained-release supplement can provide nutrients for only up to 12 hours - the time needed for food to traverse the stomach and small intestine. For this reason, even a sustained-release supplement should be taken more than once a day.

Suggestions for Comparing
Multi-Vitamin and Mineral Supplements

Most multi-vitamin supplements contain vitamins A,C,D,E, and some of the B-complex vitamins. Many contain essential minerals as well. But many are incomplete formulations and cannot be expected to provide complete nutritional protection for the body.

When purchasing health supplements, be quality-conscious. We suggest that you choose natural health supplements as much as possible. Many manufacturers include synthetic or chemical forms of vitamins (for example, dl-alpha tocopherol) and synthetic minerals such as iron in the form of ferrous sulphate. Many synthetic nutrients inhibit the absorption of nutrients in our food. For example, enriched foods that contain ferrous sulfate as iron inhibit the absorption of natural Vitamin E. Some manufacturers also use synthetic binders, fillers, and other excipients for their supplements as well as chemical colorings and flavorings. Many of these unnatural ingredients can cause allergic reactions and other problems. For the best assurance of quality health supplements and other natural medicinal aids, we suggest that you visit your health or natural food store or any of the other vitamin distributors that sell high quality health supplements.

Most forms of vitamins and minerals do not cause reactions with drugs or other medicines. They will in fact be helpful, since many drugs can deplete the body of nutrients. After being on a good total health program for some time, people who are presently taking medications should consult their physician to determine whether they may have less need for them, and thus have their prescriptions reduced.

Following are important features you should watch for when choosing the best supplement for you and your family:

1. Sustained release and divided dosage.

2. Adequate levels of all B vitamins: B1, B2, B3, B6, choline, inositol and para-aminobenzoic acid (at least 20 mg/day), B12 (30 mcg/day), biotin (200 mcg/day), and folic acid (400 mcg/day).

3. Adequate chromium (100-200 mcg/day) in the yeast or amino acid chelate form.

4. Adequate selenium (50-100 mcg/day) in the yeast or amino acid chelate form.

5. Adequate copper; a zinc-to-copper ratio of 10 or less. Example: for 20 mg zinc, at least .5 to 2 mg of copper.

6. The full complement of minerals: calcium, magnesium, potassium, iron, zinc, copper, manganese, chromium, selenium, iodine.

7. Natural formulations of vitamins and minerals.

For determining the best buy among otherwise comparable brands, and potencies, compare the cost per day for the number of tablets to be taken. Comparing the price per bottle or the price per tablet can be very misleading. For about the cost of just one soft drink per day, you should be able to establish an effective regimen that provides adequate amounts of all essential vitamins and minerals necessary to your Health Maintenance Program.

Vitamin-Mineral Information Guide

Vitamins and Minerals are essential nutrients needed for good health. The following chart provides basic information on what these nutrients are and why they are important.

KEY:
IU International Units
MG Milligrams
MCG Micrograms
RDA Recommended Daily Allowance
SDR Supplemental Dosage Recommendation

● **RDA** - Recommended Dietary Allowances are based upon recommendations of the National Academy of Sciences for healthy persons with no previous deficiencies.

● **SDR** - Supplemental Dosage Recommendations are amounts suggested to help prevent and overcome nutritional deficiencies, especially in conjunction with a good diet, plenty of exercise and a healthful lifestyle.

● Individual B Vitamin Supplements should be accompanied by a B-Complex or Multi Vitamin-Mineral Supplement.

● Pregnant women should supplement their diet in the low range of the SDR of most nutrients and in the high range of the SDR of the following nutrients: Folic Acid, Vitamin C, Calcium, Magnesium, Phosphorous, Iron, Iodine, B12 and B6.

● Including foods in your daily diet from the food source column should give you the RDA of that nutrient.

● For more than the RDA, you may want to take supplementary nutrients.

● 'Amino Acid Chelated' Minerals are the most easily absorbed and utilized form since this is the form into which your body has to incorporate minerals before it can use them.

● When meat is mentioned as a food source, lean and non-processed meats should be your first choice.

● Supplementary nutrients are best utilized when taken at the beginning of your meal.

VITAMINS

NUTRIENTS	RDA/SDR LEVELS	BEST FOOD SOURCES	DEPLETION FACTORS	BODY PARTS AND FUNCTIONS AIDED	DEFICIENCY SYMPTOMS AND BENEFICIAL USES
Vit. A - Retinol and **Beta Carotene** - Most effective with C, D, E, F, B-Complex, Calcium, Phosphorous, Zinc	RDA 5000-6000 IU SDR 10000-25000 IU Toxicity - 50000 IU Symptoms - hair loss No toxicity for beta carotene	Yellow, Orange, and Dark Green Vegetables and Fruits, Liver, Lemon Grass, Eggs, Whole Milk, Fish Liver Oil Capsules, or Beta Carotene Tablets	Caffeine, Alcohol, Mineral Oil, Excess Iron, Tobacco, Ultra-violet Rays, Birth Control Pills	Eyes, Health of Skin, Mucous Membranes, Hair and Bone Growth, Resistance to Infection, Teeth, Gums, Pregnancy & Lactation, Anti-oxidant	Night Blindness, Itch-ing Eyes, Susceptibility to Colds, Infections and Viruses, Sinus and Respiratory Problems, Asthma, Bronchitis, Al-lergies, Cystitis, Dry Skin, Eczema, Psoria-sis, Blemishes, Acne, Lack of Appetite, Fa-tigue. Beta Carotene helps lower risk of cancer, especially of the lungs.
B-Complex - All of the **B Vitamin Family** Best to take all B Vitamins Together	SDR 10-60 mg	Nutritional Yeast, Liver, Whole Grains, Brown Rice, Meat, Eggs	Caffeine, Alcohol, Sugars, Tobacco, Perspiration	Energy, Food Metabolism and Digestion, Intestinal Health, Growth, Healthy Blood Formation, Muscle Maintenance	Stress, Nerve Disor-ders, Fatigue, Head-ache, Hypoglycemia, Anemia, Allergies, Acne, Dry Skin, Insom-nia, Dry or Falling Hair, Menstrual Difficulties, Nausea, High Choles-terol, Constipation, Digestive Problems

Vitamin	RDA / SDR	Food Sources	Robbers	Functions	Deficiency Symptoms
B-1 **Thiamine** - Most effective with C, E, B-2, B Complex, Manganese, Sulphur	RDA 1-1.5 mg SDR 10-60 mg	Whole Wheat, Brown Rice, Other Whole Grains, Molasses, Raw Clams, Liver, Legumes, Nuts, Fish, Poultry, Germ and Bran of Rice, Wheat and Corn, Nutritional Yeast, Milk, Sunflower Seeds	Stress, Tobacco, Caffeine, Fever, Alcohol, Antibiotics, Surgery, Sugar	Nervous System, Energy, Brain, Growth, Muscles, Heart, Digestion, Food Metabolism, Intestinal Health, Mouth, Ears, Appetite, Blood Building, Circulation, Learning	Stress, Irritability, Nervousness, Depression, Fatigue, Noise Sensitivity, Illness, Diarrhea, Constipation, Indigestion, Anemia, General Weakness, Poor Appetite, Impaired Growth
B-2 **Riboflavin** - Most effective with B-Complex, B-6, C, Niacin	RDA 1.2-1.7 mg SDR 10-60 mg	Whole Wheat, Brown Rice, Other Whole Grains, Molasses, Liver, Lean Meat, Milk, Cheese, Nutritional Yeast, Nuts, Legumes (Peas and Beans), Bran of Rice, Wheat and Corn, Egg Yolk, Avocado, Sunflower and Sesame Seeds	Alcohol, Sugar, Tobacco, Caffeine	Healthy Eyes, Hair, Skin and Mouth, Food Metabolism, Red Blood and Antibody Formation, Oxygenation of Cells, Growth	Cracks and Sores at Corners of Mouth, Sore Tongue, Athletes Foot, Acne, Oily Face, Poor Growth, Poor Vision, Nervousness, Itching Eyes, Cataracts, Stress, Indigestion, Baldness
B-3 **Niacin or Niacinamide** Most Effective with B-Complex, C, B-1, B-2, Phosphorous	RDA 13-19 mg SDR 20-500 mg (Niacinamide Form Minimizes Flushing of Skin)	Nutritional Yeast, Whole Grains, Rice, Bran, Prunes, Apricots, Citrus, Nuts, Cayenne, Lean Meat, Fish, Poultry, Mushrooms, Green Vegetables, Beans	Stress, Infection, Sugar, Caffeine, Alcohol, Antibiotics, Trauma	Food Metabolism (Especially Sugar), Nervous System, Digestion, Adrenal Glands, Sex Hormones, Skin, Tongue, Improves Circulation	High Blood Pressure, Poor Circulation, Cold Extremities, Leg Cramps, Migraine Headaches, Depression, Nervousness, Fatigue, Pellagra, Acne, Skin Eruptions, Poor Digestion, Canker Sores, Halitosis-Bad Breath

NUTRIENTS	RDA/SDR LEVELS	BEST FOOD SOURCES	DEPLETION FACTORS	BODY PARTS AND FUNCTIONS AIDED	DEFICIENCY SYMPTOMS AND BENEFICIAL USES
B-5 **Pantothenic Acid** Most Effective With B Complex, B-12, B-6, C, Folic Acid, Biotin, Sulphur	RDA 4-7 mg SDR 40-100 mg	Whole Grains, Wheat Germs, Mushrooms, Eggs, Liver, Salmon, Nutritional Yeast, Molasses, Legumes (Beans & Peas)	Stress, Caffeine, Alcohol, Antibiotics, Meat, Insecticides	Adrenal Glands (Stress Resistance), Digestion, Food Metabolism, Skin, Nerves, Growth, Energy, Convulsion, Antibody Formation, Vitamin Utilization	Stress, Weak Adrenal Glands, Allergies, Nervousness, Duodenal Ulcers, Exhaustion, Arthritis, Dizziness, Digestive Disorders, Graying Hair, Hair Loss, Hypoglycemia, Retarded Growth, Premature Aging, Skin Abnormalities
B-6 **Pyridoxine** - Most Effective With B-Complex, F, C, Potassium, Magnesium	RDA 2-2.2 mg SDR 10-60 mg	Whole Wheat, Brown Rice, Other Whole Grains, Molasses, Liver, Bran of Rice, Wheat and Corn, Nutritional Yeast, Milk, Egg Yolk, Fish, Cabbage, Beets, Green Leafy Vegetables	X-Rays, Caffeine, Alcohol, Tobacco, Birth Control Pills	Nerves, Blood, Antibodies, Muscles, Skin Health, Sodium-Potassium Balance, Food Metabolism and Digestion, Weight Control, Red Blood Cells	Stress, Nervousness, Depression, Insomnia, Irritability, Dizziness, Overweight, Diuretic, High Cholesterol, Atherosclerosis, Hardening of Arteries, Acne, Hypoglycemia, Anemia, Premenstrual Tension, Nausea in Pregnancy, Bursitis

Vitamin	RDA / SDR	Food Sources	Enemies	Functions	Deficiency Symptoms
B-12 Cobalamin - Most Effective With B-Complex, C, Potassium, Folic Acid, Calcium	RDA 3 mcg SDR 20-100 mcg	Cheese, Fish, Milk, Cottage Cheese, Pork, Liver, Beef, Eggs, Soy Tempeh, Spirulina, Kelp, Pollen, Comfrey, (Supplement may be necessary for strict Vegetarians)	Laxatives, Caffeine, Alcohol, Tobacco	Nervous System, Helps Iron Build Red Blood, Growth, Appetite, Food Metabolism, Cell Longevity	Pernicious Anemia, General Weakness, Fatigue, Loss of Appetite, Nervousness, Allergies, Stress, Shingles, Nerve Degeneration, Overweight, Walking & Speaking Difficulties
Pangamic Acid - Sometimes called **Vitamin B-15**. Most effective with B-Complex, C & E	RDA 10 mg SDR 10-60 mg	Whole Grains, Nutritional Yeast, Sunflower, Sesame, Pumpkin Seeds, Brown Rice	Alcohol, Caffeine	Heart, Respiration, Breathing, Detoxification, Cell Oxygenation, Glandular and Nervous System Stimulation	Shortness of Breath, Shallow Breathing, Fatigue, Emphysema, Respiration Impairment, Oxygenation to Heart, Heart Disease, Impaired Circulation, Glandular Disorders, Carbon Monoxide Poisoning (from Pollution)
Biotin - Part of B-Complex - Most Effective with B-Complex, C, B-12, Sulphur, Folic Acid	RDA 150-300 mcg SDR 100-200 mcg	Eggs, Liver, Whole Wheat, Brown Rice, Other Whole Grains, Nutritional Yeast, Lentils, Sardines, Poultry	Oxidation, Alcohol, Caffeine, Antibiotics, Raw Egg White	Food Metabolism, Hair and Cell Growth, B-Complex Utilization, Fatty Acid Production, Conversion of Nucleic Acids	Muscle Pain, Exhaustion, Depression, Hair Loss, Dry or Graying Hair, Dermatitis, Poor Appetite

NUTRIENTS	RDA/SDR LEVELS	BEST FOOD SOURCES	DEPLETION FACTORS	BODY PARTS AND FUNCTIONS AIDED	DEFICIENCY SYMPTOMS AND BENEFICIAL USES
Inositol - part of **B-Complex Family** - Most Effective with B-Complex, C, B-1, B-2, B-12, Phosphorous, Choline, Linoleic Acid	RDA 60 mg SDR 50-300 mg	Lecithin, Whole Grains, Citrus, Nutritional Yeast, Vegetables, Liver, Molasses, Nuts, Milk, Meat, Eggs, Wheat Germ	Sugar, Caffeine, Alcohol, Antibiotics	Reduces Cholesterol, Metabolism of Fats and Cholesterol, Hair Growth, Brain, Eye Membranes, Weight Control	Sleeplessness, Eczema, Hair Loss, Eye Problems, High Cholesterol, Atherosclerosis, Constipation, Overweight
Choline - part of **B Complex Family** - Most Effective with B-Complex, A, Linoleic Acid, Inositol	RDA 60 mg SDR 50-250 mg	Eggs, Wheat Germ, Legumes, Liver, Soybeans, Lecithin, Nutritional Yeast	Sugar, Alcohol, Caffeine, Insecticide	Hair, Thymus Gland, Gall Bladder and Liver Regulation, Weight Control, Metabolism of Fats, Nerve Transmissions, Healthy Arteries, Reduces Cholesterol	High Cholesterol, Hardening of the Arteries (Atherosclerosis), High Blood Pressure, Cirrhosis of Liver, Hair Loss, Stomach Ulcers, Gallstones, Ringing in Ears, Dizziness, Overweight
Folic Acid - part of **B-Complex Family** - Most Effective with B-Complex, B-12, C, Biotin, Pantothenic Acid	RDA 400 mcg SDR 400-1200 mcg	Green Leafy Vegetables, Nutritional Yeast, Tuna, Salmon, Oysters, Whole Grains, Mushrooms, Liver, Milk, Nuts, Dry Beans	Stress, Alcohol, Caffeine, Tobacco, Streptomycin, Birth Control Pills	Red Blood Cells, Body Growth and Reproduction, Protein Metabolism, Hydrochloric Acid Production, Healthy Glands and Liver	Anemia, B-12 Deficiency, Fatigue, Slow Growth, Menstrual Problems, Birth Defects, Reproductive Disorders, Diarrhea, Stress, Graying Hair, Loss of Hair

Nutrient	Dosage	Food Sources	Depleted By	Benefits	Deficiency Symptoms
PABA - Para Amino Benzoic Acid - Most Effective with B-Complex, C, Folic Acid	RDA 10 mg SDR 10-100 mg	Green Vegetables, Wheat Germ, Liver, Nutritional Yeast, Molasses, Milk, Meat	Caffeine, Alcohol, Sulfonamides	Skin, Hair, Intestines, Protein Metabolism, Muscles, Hair Color Restoration, Natural Sunscreen	Fatigue (especially after muscle use), Graying Hair, Dark Skin Spots, Poor Intestinal Activity, Folic Acid Production, Anemia, Headaches
C - Ascorbic Acid - Most Effective with All Vitamins, Minerals and Bioflavonoids	RDA 50-100 mg SDR 250-3000 mg Intake from 5000-15000 mg may cause diarrhea in some individuals	Fresh Fruits and Vegetables, including Alfalfa Sprouts	Stress, Alcohol, Caffeine, Tobacco, Mercury, Fever, Overcooking, Aspirin, Cortizone, Pasteurization, Pollution, Sulfonomides, Perspiration	Teeth, Gums, Bones, Blood and Blood Vessels, Infection Resistance, Collagen Production, Iron Assimilation, Wound Healing, Vitamin Protection (Anti-Oxidant), Aids Longevity, Adrenals	Susceptibility to Infections (Colds, Viruses, Flu, etc.), Allergies, Stress, Anemia, Blood Vessel Rupture (Hemorrhoids, Bruising, Varicose Veins, Nose Bleeds), Bleeding Gums, Dental Cavities, Strengthen Skin Tissue, Atherosclerosis, Cystitis, Arthritis
D-3 (Natural Form) - **Cholecalciferol** - Most Effective with A, C, F, Phosphorous, Calcium, Choline	RDA 200-400 IU SDR 400-800 IU	Sunshine, Fish Liver Oil, Egg Yolk, Liver, Salmon, Tuna, Herring, Cod Liver Oil (Synthesized Form-D2 is found in Milk)	Mineral Oil	Bone and Teeth Formation, Calcium Absorption, Phosphorous Assimilation, Nerves, Thyroid, Blood Clotting	Soft Bones and Teeth, Bone Disease, Tooth Decay, Gum Disease, Nervousness, Poor Metabolism, Muscular Weakness, Diarrhea, Eczema, Psoriasis, Arthritis

NUTRIENTS	RDA/SDR LEVELS	BEST FOOD SOURCES	DEPLETION FACTORS	BODY PARTS AND FUNCTIONS AIDED	DEFICIENCY SYMPTOMS AND BENEFICIAL USES
E - D-Alpha Tocopherol (not DI-Alpha) - Most Effective with B Complex, A, C, F, Maganese, Selenium	RDA 8-10 IU SDR 50-800 IU Older persons and those with heart problems should begin with a low osage	Whole Grains, Wheat Germ Oil, Cold Pressed Vegetable Oil, Seeds, Nuts, Soybeans, Eggs, Organ Meats, Dark Green Vegetables	Ultraviolet, Oxidation, Rancid Fat and Oil, Mineral Oil, Chlorine, Birth Control Pills, Air Pollution, Inorganic Iron (Ferrous Sulphate and Ferrous Chloride)	Blood Flow to Heart, Circulation, Anti-oxidant (slows aging and preserves fats and oils). Retards Blood Clotting, Reproduction, Cell Oxygenation, Prostate, Blood and Capillary Maintenance, Muscle and Nerve Maintenance, Healthy Hair and Skin, Lung Protection	Heart Diseases, Strokes, Atheroscler-osis, High Cholesterol, Calcium Deposits, Muscular Dystrophy, Enlarged Prostate, Impotency, Sterility, Menopausal & Men-strual Problems, Mis-carriage, Cystitis, Thrombosis, Phlebitis, Varicose Veins. **Antiox-idant** - Protects Lungs from Pollution. **External** - Burns, Scars, Wrinkles, Wounds, Warts
Unsaturated Fatty Acids - Often **Called Vitamin F** - Most Effective with E, A, D, C, Phosphorous	RDA 2 Tbsp. SDR 10% of Total Calories	Wheat Germ and Vegetable Oils, Seeds, Cod Liver Oil	Radiation, Oxidation, Mineral Oil	Health of Skin and Hair, Sex Organs, Glands, Mucous Membranes, Growth, Prevent Cholesterol Buildup, Lubrication and Resilience of Skin	Dry Skin Disorders, Eczema, Psoriasis, Acne, Dry Hair, Dandruff, High Cholesterol, Heart Disease, Rheumatoid Arthritis, Gallstones, Diarrhea, Menopause (Natural Hormones)

Nutrient	RDA / SDR	Food Sources	Enemies	Functions	Deficiency Symptoms
Vit. K **Phylloquinone**	RDA 300 mcg SDR 100-300 mcg	Kelp, Alfalfa, Green Vegetables, Other Green Plants, Eggs, Milk, Cauliflower, Soy Beans, Polyunsaturated Oil, Yogurt	Mineral Oil, Rancid Fats, X-Rays, Antibiotics, Aspirin	Bile Absorption, Growth, Cell Longevity, Promotes Blood Coagulation, Liver Function	Hemorrhaging and Prolonged Bleeding, Hemophilia, Nosebleeds, Prolonged Menstruation, Miscarriages, and Cellular Disease
Vit. P (Rutin, Hesperidin) **Bioflavonoids** - Most Effective with C, Calcium, Magnesium	RDA 500 mg SDR 50-500 mg	Citrus, Buckwheat, Green Pepper, Black Currants, Cherries, Grapes, Onions, Garlic, Parsley, Tomato	Stress, High Fever, Alcohol, Tobacco, Aspirin, Excess Salt, Cortisone, Air Pollution	Blood Vessel and Capillary Strength, Resistance to Infection, Connective Tissue, Vit. C Utilization	Bruising, Nosebleeds, Hemorrhoids, Varicose Veins, Duodenal Ulcers, Miscarriages, Colds

MINERALS

NUTRIENTS	RDA/SDR LEVELS	BEST FOOD SOURCES	DEPLETION FACTORS	BODY PARTS AND FUNCTIONS AIDED	DEFICIENCY SYMPTOMS AND BENEFICIAL USES
Calcium - Most Effective with A, C, D, F, Magnesium, Phosphorous, Iron, Manganese, Iron, Hydrochloric Acid	RDA 800-1200 mg SDR 800-1500 mg	Dairy, Dark Green Vegetables, Sesame Seeds and Sesame Tahini, Legumes, Tofu, Nuts, Seaweed	Stress, Lack of: Exercise, HCL, Magnesium, or Vitamin D	Bones, Teeth, Heart Rhythm, Endurance, Blood Clotting, Iron Utilization and Relaxation of Nerves	Sore Muscles, Back-ache, Muscle Cramps, Menstrual Cramps, Pre-Menstrual Tension, Menopause Problems, Brittle Nails and Bones, Bone Disease, Nerve Problems, Insomnia, Heart Palpitations, Arthritis, Tooth and Gum Problems
Chromium	RDA 50-200 mcg SDR 100-300 mcg	Nutritional Yeast, Whole Grains, Clams, Corn Oil, Liver, Lean Meat	Air Pollution, Sugar Metabolism	Blood Sugar Levels, Increases Effect of Insulin, Circulatory System, Metabolism of Glucose (Energy), Thyroid and Adrenal Glands	Glucose Intolerance, Hypoglycemia, Diabetes, Atherosclerosis

Nutrient	RDA / SDR	Sources	Antagonists	Functions	Deficiency
Copper - Most Effective with Zinc, Cobalt, Iron, C	RDA 2-3 mg SDR .5-2 mg	Seafood, Seaweed, Nuts, Raisins, Green Leafy Vegetables, Soybeans, Legumes, Whole Grains, Liver	Excess Zinc, Aspirin	Enzymes, Elastin, Red Blood, Hair and Skin Color, Bone Formation, Iron Absorption, Healing Process	Pernicious anemia, General Weakness, Skin Sores, Respiratory Problems, Retarded Growth
Iodine	RDA 150 mcg SDR 100-225 mcg	Wheat Germ, Fish, Kelp Tablets, Seaweed, Mushroom, Garlic	None	Thyroid, Metabolic Rate, Fat Metabolism, Energy Production, Hair, Skin, Nails, Teeth, Growth, Speech, Mental Development	Goiter, Hypothyroidism, Hyperthyroidism, Obesity, Atherosclerosis, Cold Extremities, Irritability, Dry Hair
Iron - Most Effective With C, B12, B6, Folic Acid, Copper, Phosphorous, Calcium, HCL Acid	RDA 10-18 mg SDR 15-50 mg	Liver, Wheat Germ, Oysters, Molasses, Green Leafy Vegetables, Legumes, Poultry, Fish, Eggs, Dried Fruit, Whole Grains	Coffee, Bleeding, Excess Zinc and Phosphorous, Diarrhea, Over-cooking	Hemoglobin, Myoglobin, Protein Metabolism, Energy, Oxygen to Muscle Cells, Stress, Disease Resistance, Growth, Health of Skin, Nails, Teeth and Bones	Anemia, Blood Loss, Fatigue, Pale Skin, Menstrual Problems, Brittle Nails, Breathing Difficulties, Constipation, Colitis

NUTRIENTS	RDA/SDR LEVELS	DEPLETION FACTORS	BEST FOOD SOURCES	BODY PARTS AND FUNCTIONS AIDED	DEFICIENCY SYMPTOMS AND BENEFICIAL USES
Magnesium - Most Effective With C, D, B6, Calcium, Phosphorous, Protein	RDA 300-400 mg SDR 300-500 mg	Alcohol, Diuretics, High Cholesterol	Dark Green Vegetables, Whole Grains, Wheat Germ, Fish, Seaweed, Molasses, Nuts, Legumes, Seeds	Nerves, Calcium and Vit. C Absorption, Bones, Arteries, Muscles, Teeth, Heart, Memory, Acid-Alkaline Balance, Blood Sugar Metabolism (Energy)	Calcium Deposits, Kidney Stones, Arteriosclerosis, Heart Problems, Blood Clots, Nervousness, Irritability, Exhaustion, Muscle Twitches, Confusion, Convulsions (Epilepsy), Tooth Decay, Soft Bones (Osteoporosis), Stomach Acid (as Antacid)
Manganese - Most Effective With B1, E, Calcium, Phosphorous	RDA 2.5-5 mg SDR 5-50 mg	Excess Phosphorous and Calcium	Whole Grains, Buckwheat, Eggs, Green Vegetables, Carrot, Celery, Beet, Legumes, Nuts, Pineapples, Liver, Bran	Enzyme Activation, Fats and Carbohydrate Metabolism, Bones, Sex Hormones, Growth, Spleen, Brain, Pancreas, Heart	Dizziness, Diabetes (Glucose Intolerance), Loss of Muscular Coordination, Glandular Disorders, Hearing Loss or Noises, Male Impotence and Sterility

Mineral	RDA / SDR	Sources	Depleters	Functions	Deficiency Symptoms
Phosphorous - Most Effective With A, D, Calcium, HCL Acid, F, Iron, Protein	RDA 800-1200 mg SDR 50-150 mg	Lean Meat, Fish, Poultry, Eggs, Whole Grains, Nuts, Dairy, Legumes, Seeds, Seaweeds, Green Vegetables	Antacids, Sugar, Excess of: Fats, Aluminum, Magnesium, Iron	Bone and Tooth Formation, Cell Growth & Repair, Brain, Nerve and Muscle Activity, Vitamin Utilization, Energy, Food Metabolism, Calcium and Sugar Metabolism, Heart Contractions	Bone Disease, Nervous Disorders, Stress, Weakness, Fatigue, Tooth and Gum Disorders, Stunted Growth, Weight Problems, Irregular Breathing
Potassium - Most Effective With B6, Sodium	RDA 1500-2500 mg SDR 100-500 mg	Whole Grains, Bananas, Milk, Prunes, Raisins, Figs, Seaweed, Green Vegetables, Legumes, Fish, Seeds, Potatoes	Diuretics, Caffeine, Alcohol, Laxatives, Stress, Cortisone, Excess Salt & Sugar, Vomiting	Kidney Functions, Heartbeat, Muscle Contraction, Skin, Proper Alkalinity, Enzyme Reactions, Nerves, Potassium-Sodium Balance	Irregular Heartbeat, Toxic Kidneys, Nervousness, Insomnia, Dry Skin, Acne, Muscle Damage, General Weakness, High Blood Pressure
Selenium (bound to yeast) - Most Effective with Vitamin E	RDA 50-200 mcg SDR 50-200 mcg Toxicity - 500 mcg	Nutritional Yeast, Eggs, Garlic, Whole Grains, Broccoli, Onions, Tomato, Tuna, Seaweed, Herring, Seeds, Mushrooms	Mercury Poisoning	Tissue Elasticity, Scalp, Metabolism, Growth, Antioxidant, Fertility, Immune System, Neutralizes Carcinogens, Pancreatic Function	Premature Aging, Insomnia, Inflexibility, Dandruff, Arteriosclerosis, Impaired Male Sexual Function

NUTRIENTS	RDA/SDR LEVELS	BEST FOOD SOURCES	DEPLETION FACTORS	BODY PARTS AND FUNCTIONS AIDED	DEFICIENCY SYMPTOMS AND BENEFICIAL USES
Sulphur - Most Effective With B Complex	RDA None Stated SDR Not Established	Eggs, Dairy, Fish, Lean Meats, Nuts, Wheat Germ, Legumes, Sprouts, Seaweed, Cabbage Family	Unknown	Health of Skin, Hair, Nails, Cartilage, Cell Respiration, Liver Elimination	Flatulence (poor fat digestion), Dermatitis, Eczema, Psoriasis, Brittle Nails and Hair, Wound Healing
Zinc - Most Effective With A, Copper, Calcium, Phosphorous	RDA 15 mg SDR 20-50 mg	Liver, Whole Grains, Eggs, Mushrooms, Nuts, Bran, Leafy Vegetables, Pumpkin and Sunflower Seeds, Fish, Nutritional Yeast, Soybeans	Lack of Phosphorous, Alcohol, Excess Calcium	Sex Organs, Brain, Hair, Prostate, Skin, DNA-RNA Synthesis, Wound and Burn Healing, Digestion and Metabolism, B Complex Utilization	Prostate Problems, Loss of Taste, Poor Appetite, Wound Healing, Sterility, Fatigue, Retarded Growth, Diabetes, Infertility, Delayed Sexual Maturity, White Spots Under Fingernails

Mineral	RDA / SDR	Sources	Depleted By / Function	Function	Deficiency Symptoms
Sodium - Most Effective with Vit. D and Potassium	RDA 1100-3000 mg SDR None	Salt, Dairy Products, Seafood and Seaweed, Meat, Poultry, Green Vegetables	Chlorine, Lack of Potassium, Diuretic	Normal Cellular Fluid Level, Osmotic Cell Pressure, Proper Muscle Contraction, Alkaline Balance, Blood, Lymph	Weight Loss, Alkalosis, Muscle Cramps, Dehydration, Dry Tongue. **Excess Symptoms:** High Blood Pressure, Poor Protein Absorption, Fluid Retention (Edema), Thirst, Insomnia, Nervousness, Irritability
Chlorine - (Chloride) Excess Destroys Vit. E, Intestinal Flora	RDA 500 mg SDR None	Potassium Chloride or Table Salt, Seaweed, Rye, Oats, Salt Water Fish		Protein Digestion, Liver Cleansing, Hydrochloric Acid Production, Acid-Alkaline Balance, Osmotic Cell Pressure, Destroys Bad Bacteria & Stomach Parasites	Hair and Tooth Loss, Impaired Digestion, Poor Muscle Contraction

NOTE: The symptoms noted on these pages could occur only when the daily intake of the vitamins mentioned has been less than the minimum daily requirement over a prolonged period. These non-specific symptoms do not alone prove a nutritional deficiency but may be caused by any great number of conditions or may have functional causes. If these symptoms persist they may indicate a condition other than a vitamin or mineral deficiency. It is recommended that any unusual or prolonged symptoms be looked into by a competent professional.

For any treatment or diagnosis of illness see your physician. This chart is not intended to be diagnostic or prescriptive, but is for information purposes only. Individuals allergic to certain dietary supplements should consult a physician for advice.

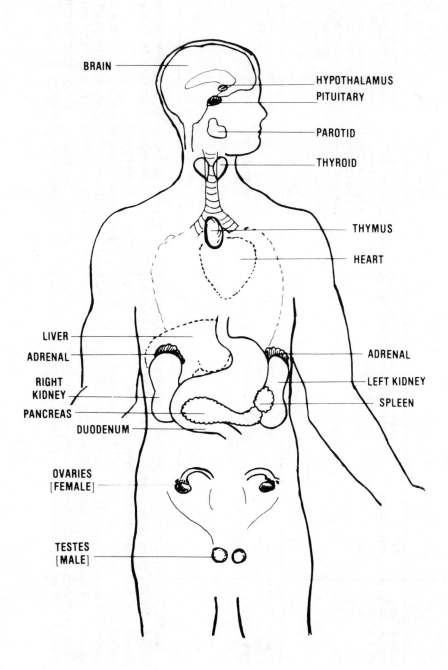

BRAIN

HYPOTHALAMUS
PITUITARY

PAROTID

THYROID

THYMUS

HEART

LIVER
ADRENAL

RIGHT
KIDNEY

PANCREAS

DUODENUM

ADRENAL

LEFT KIDNEY

SPLEEN

OVARIES
[FEMALE]

TESTES
[MALE]

YOUR BODY'S GLANDS AND ORGANS

The **Glands** and **Organs** of the body are responsible for many bodily functions. They play a major role in growth, development, metabolism, and many other activities. Glands can often become weak, sluggish, or erratic. One reason for their weakness may be from differences in inherited physiological capabilities. Thus everyone's requirements and needs differ. This is biochemical individuality. Malfunctions of glands or organs can also result from lack of nutrients, overstimulation, the process of aging, or some other form of abuse to the body. Stress, anemia, low blood sugar, impaired sexual functioning and many other problems could result.

The health of your glands and organs can be improved with supplements of the specific glandular or organ concentrate. Certain factors in their concentrates can be utilized by the particular gland or organ in your body to improve its functioning.

The health of glands and organs can also be supported by good nutrition, which includes a good diet and perhaps vitamin supplementation. Since many glands influence and interact with other glands, a multiple gland or organ supplement can be a good basis for support. And of course improving your entire lifestyle would not only improve the general health of your body, but also the specific glands and organs.

There are nutritional supplements available which are made from the extracts of glands and organs of healthy New Zealand range-fed animals which are not exposed to pesticides, herbicides, synthetic hormones, etc. These contain factors that can nourish the particular gland or organ in your body. They are formulated in a liquid base to be taken under the tongue to ensure better and quicker assimilation and to avoid destruction of the nutrients in the stomach. These products are developed through the methods of homeopathy, a formal branch of medicine based on the principle that 'like heals like.' This **Law of Similars** also applies to modern allergenic and vaccination therapy. If you would like more information on how and where to obtain these products, please write to us.

The **Thymus** gland creates white blood cells (lymphocytes), that in turn manufacture antibodies that assist the immune system in combating disease and infection.

The **Pituitary** gland aids proper functioning of the thyroid, adrenal, testes and ovary glands. It also secretes a growth hormone that assists in controlling metabolism, as well as other hormones that influence kidney function, blood pressure and smooth muscle action.

The **Thyroid** gland regulates the rate of metabolism of your body, which is reflected in how much energy you feel and how efficiently you utilize food calories. The thyroid also influences physical and mental growth, increased circulatory flow, and the prevention of an accumulation of calcium in the blood stream.

The **Kidneys** function as filters of waste products, toxins and other foreign substances from the urine. They are also responsible for maintaining fluid levels, salt levels and acid-alkaline balance in the body. If the kidneys become overloaded with toxic substances they can be weakened or even damaged. Kidney stones, infections and even hypertension can damage the kidneys.

The **Ovaries** in women secrete hormones that are responsible for sexual characteristics of the female, including sex organs, breast enlargement, uterus, etc. The ovaries maintain a regular cycle of estrogen and progesterone, as well as being responsible for the regular production of ova or eggs. In women, low levels of female hormones can result in the degeneration of the reproductive system as well as in the reduction of secondary sexual characteristics.

The **Testes** (orchic) in men produce the hormones that control the development of primary and secondary sexual characteristics as well as sexual impulses of the male. They are also responsible for the manufacture of sperm, the male reproductive cells.

The **Adrenal** glands are sometimes known as the stress glands. They protect the body from stress by producing hormones that help to counter stress. Some hormones help regulate blood sugar levels (energy levels), while others regulate the amount of certain minerals in the body, especially sodium and potassium. The adrenals produce steroid hormones, including cortisone, that help reduce inflammation, thus allowing the body to heal with less pain and discomfort. Diseases such as arthritis can be aided by healthy adrenals. Steroid hormones also help to regulate the immune system, thus helping the body resist infections, allergies, etc. Androgens produced in the adrenal gland aid in building and properly distributing muscle tissue. With natural adrenal gland supplements, athletes could avoid harmful synthetic hormones and still develop well-proportioned, healthy muscles. Properly functioning adrenals will keep aging spots to a minimum, as well as minimizing menopausal symptons by maintaining adequate hormone levels. Vitamin C and the B vitamin Pantothenic Acid support the adrenal glands.

The **Pancreas** produces insulin, necessary to change glucose (blood sugar) to energy. The pancreas can be weakened from the overproduction of insulin. Eventually it may produce too little insulin, which can lead to diabetic tendencies. Another hormone regulates the transformation of stored sugars (glycogen) back to blood sugar as needed. An insufficient amount of this hormone can result in hypoglycemic effects. The pancreas is also important in the digestion of protein, fat and carbohydrates in the intestinal tract where it secretes several digestive enzymes.

CARDIOVASCULAR SYSTEM

This system consists of the heart, the arteries, veins and capillaries. Its blood circulatory functions are three-fold. First, it carries used blood to the lungs to be purified and oxygenated at several locations enroute. Secondly, it carries the clean, oxygenated blood back from the lungs to the rest of the body. And third, it picks up nutrients along the way and feeds them to wherever they are needed.

The heart is responsible for pumping blood through your body. The entire cardiovascular system can become sluggish as a result of poor nutritional practices. This sluggishness can cause a buildup of cholesterol and calcium in your vessels and arteries. Poor circulation results, forcing the heart to work overtime in pumping blood through your arteries. As a result, your heart can be weakened or damaged from stroke or other heart disease, including high blood pressure.

The more exercise you do the stronger your heart becomes, and in turn the easier it is for the heart to pump your blood. Exercise also helps your blood to remove toxins and wastes as well as lowering the amount of harmful deposits in your bloodstream. All of this then, will improve your blood circulation and nourish your body tissues, organs and cells with more nutrients.

The main thing we can all do nutritionally to remain free of heart problems is to limit our intake of fats.

The nutrients most important for the nutritional support of the cardiovascular system are Vitamin E, Lecithin (a source of choline), B complex, Vitamin C and the minerals calcium, magnesium and potassium. Of these, Vitamin E is the most important to oxygenate the blood and improve circulation, magnesium is necessary to keep calcium deposits from forming, and choline helps to prevent cholesterol deposits. Heart tissue concentrate would also be helpful for the nourishment of heart muscle. It can improve heart muscle function, stabilize rhythm and restore tonicity.

Some Risk Factors Associated with Heart Disease

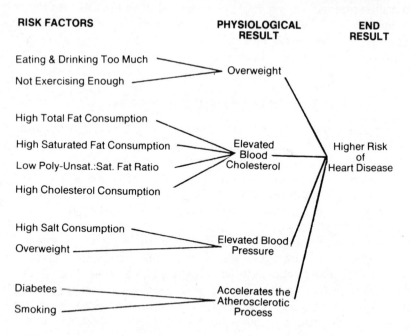

RISK FACTORS **PHYSIOLOGICAL RESULT** **END RESULT**

Eating & Drinking Too Much
Not Exercising Enough
→ Overweight

High Total Fat Consumption
High Saturated Fat Consumption
Low Poly-Unsat.:Sat. Fat Ratio
High Cholesterol Consumption
→ Elevated Blood Cholesterol

High Salt Consumption
Overweight
→ Elevated Blood Pressure

Diabetes
Smoking
→ Accelerates the Atherosclerotic Process

→ Higher Risk of Heart Disease

RESPIRATORY SYSTEM (LUNGS)

The lungs are the respiratory organs of the body and are responsible for the intake of oxygen. Oxygen is important for our metabolism, energy level, digestion, healthy blood and various other functions.

Our lungs are vital for the exchange of oxygen and carbon dioxide. They help to eliminate carbon dioxide — the waste product from that exchange process. This whole process can be made much more efficient by getting adequate exercise.

Nutrients most needed to aid the health of your lungs and oxygenation of your blood are Vitamins E, C and A. These nutrients keep oxygen from being destroyed. Lung tissue concentrate can also help to nourish damaged lungs.

NERVOUS SYSTEM AND BRAIN

The nervous system is controlled by the brain. Your nervous system controls your mental activity and your nerve energy. Your brain needs to be nourished just like any other part of your body.

The health of the entire nervous system can be aided nutritionally by the Vitamin B complex, that is, all of the B vitamins. Other nutrients that nourish the nerves are Vitamins A, fatty acids, calcium, magnesium and potassium. Brain tissue concentrate can also be beneficial by providing substances necessary to normal nerve and brain functioning.

Most importantly you need to keep a good positive mental attitude, free from stress at all times. A good diet is also very important, as well as enough rest and relaxation to regenerate your nerve energy.

HERBS

Many people today are finding herbs to be beneficial nutritional and medicinal aids. To some people these are strange new products, but to others, herbs have been around their entire lives. Herbs have been used as medicines for centuries. Herbal products today have been formulated to provide as much safety to consumers as possible. They are high in certain vitamins, minerals and a variety of other health-promoting constituents.

Many herbs can be obtained as teas or as supplements either individually or in combinations formulated to help you with particular health problems. Many studies have shown herbs to be very effective in the treatment of many disease. They are also safer than most drugs. However, before you begin to use herbs for particular health situations, we strongly recommend that you consult with a health professional who is very knowledgeable in their use, as herbs can have a very powerful effect on your body. Hopefully it will be a good effect, but since you are using these herbs as medicines it is safer to consult someone who is very experienced with their use, and it is certainly not a good idea to rely solely on herbs to correct health problems. Instead you should concentrate on living as healthful a life as you possibly can so you won't need the herbal medicine in the first place.

There are some very tasty herbal teas that are not medicinal and make for delightful drinking on cold winter days, or iced on a hot summer day. These are available at health food stores and some grocery stores.

MEDICATION/DRUG USE

A drug is any chemical which you take in order to affect your body or mind. There is no such thing as a completely safe drug.

Anything you take into your body can have a toxic effect if taken in the wrong quantity or if you are sensitive to it. The more powerful the drug, the greater the potential for harmful effects.

Today there is an epidemic of drug misuse. Drugs include medically prescribed, over-the-counter preparations, and "recreational" or "street" drugs. Misuse includes not following directions for correct dosage, over-medicating yourself and taking drugs with alcohol or in combination with other drugs. "Recreational" or "street" drugs pose an additional threat due to questionable purity and unknown strength or concentration. Most drugs are meant to work with your body promoting the self-healing process and providing relief from a symptom. If you use them improperly, they can't do their jobs...and you'll be the loser. Misuse of drugs or medications can cause complications of pre-existing conditions, failure to improve, permanent damage to organs, and even death.

To protect yourself, read all labels carefully. Make sure you understand how much, how often, and for how long you should take any medication. Be aware of dangerous interactions with food, alcohol or other drugs. Keep up-to-date a list of all medications you take. Check this list with your physician or pharmacist to make sure none can interact in a harmful manner.

Many special medications are extremely powerful chemicals and often long-term use may be an additional risk to health. Currently, some controversy exists as to how much and for how long these drugs are to be used.

You should take antibiotics only on a short term basis when you have dental work, surgery, or if you have an accident where the skin is broken allowing infection to enter your system. Driving your car while under the influence of any type of drug that makes you drowsy, alters your mood, or slows your reaction time is a threat to your health, as well as the safety of others. Sometimes the combination of alcohol with other drugs is a particularly deadly combination. No drugs — not even aspirin — should be taken by pregnant women without the approval of a physician. Always be alert for potentially dangerous drug combinations. If you are in doubt, consult your physician or pharmacist. The best advice however, is to use all of the information we provide in this book to stay optimally healthy so you don't need medication, or at least so you can cut down on its use.

Always try to find a nutrition-minded physician who can perhaps get you well with alternative methods to medication.

CHANGING YOUR HABITS

"Habit is Habit. It is not to be flung out of the window by anyone, but coaxed downstairs a step at a time." - Mark Twain

The patterns of our daily lives — our habits — have a profound effect on our health. And as the above quotation implies, changing these patterns into ones that maximize your chances for optimum health and well-being is often a time-consuming, difficult process.

However, after reading this book, you will know the basics of good health and be ready to learn more. The first thing you can do is to make the decision to start now. Make the commitment to take responsibility for your own body. You must believe that you can and do have the ability to follow the "Laws of Health."

Decide what improvements you want to make. You might want to choose an aspect of your nutritional habits or of your lifestyle that you feel you can successfully change most easily. You should take charge of your life, take charge of your diet and your attitude, begin a good exercise program and replace stressful worry with a positive plan.

Don't feel you're a failure if you can't completely eliminate certain unhealthful aspects of your lifestyle such as smoking, alcohol, coffee and soda drinking, poor eating habits, etc. Even small improvements in health habits are significant. Healthy lifestyles are built of many small blocks. You'll be happy and pleased with even the small changes you are able to make. Depending on someone else to change your habits usually does not work.

The Steps to Self-Cure

How does anyone manage to kick a habit after years of living with it? The answer lies in self-cure. It involves three components necessary for change: an urge to quit, the belief that you can quit, and the realization that you must quit — no one can do it for you. Once you have quit, the rewards of living without the habit or addiction must be great enough to keep you free of it.

The stages of successful self-cure are remarkably similar, regardless of the habit.

(1.) **Becoming aware of what we want to change.** We need to be aware of any negative results of a bad habit as well as all the positive effects of changing the habit.

(2.) **Accumulated unhappiness about the habit.** Before a change can take place, unhappiness with the habit has to build to a point where it can't be denied or rationalized away. To break a habit or addiction, you must believe that the rewards you'll get (from not smoking, from exercising and losing weight, from cutting down on or giving up alcohol, drugs or junk foods) will surpass what you got from the habit.

(3.) **Visualization** is another very useful method that involves using your imagination to help change habits or even to help heal yourself from illness or stress. Just sit for a moment, close your eyes and relax. Then visualize or imagine yourself being healthier, happier and more alive after having removed a particular bad habit. Visualize what you want for yourself as if you are experiencing it now. Continue the visualization changing it in any way you feel may be helpful. Repeated visualizations will bring you what you want by keeping you aware of how healthy you could be and feel without certain habits.

(4.) **Moment of truth.** Various dramatic events in our lives can bring about a new way of looking at our lives — as when an alcoholic embarrasses him or herself in front of others, a cigarette smoker watching a friend die of lung cancer, etc. But most moments of truth seem to be inspired by trivial remarks or chance occurrences.

(5.) **Changing patterns.** People successful at self-cure usually make active changes in their environment — they may move away from a drug culture, become more involved in work, make new friends.

(6.) **Gaining a new identity.** Once a person gains more from a new life than from the old ways — feeling better, working better, having more fun — the old ways have no appeal.

One easy place to start is with your nutritional habits. Reduce the amount of prepared foods in your cupboard and walk to a store that carries fresh fruits and vegetables, whole grain breads and cereals and other wholesome natural foods.

Perhaps you may not be ready to change your eating habits completely or maybe you are unfamiliar with how to plan a tasty nutritious meal with less salt, meat and other foods that may be detrimental to your health. Start looking at natural food and vegetarian cookbooks for meals. We recommend several choices: **Recipes for a Small Planet, For the Love of Food, Deaf Smith Country Cookbook,** and **Laurel's Kitchen,** but there are many more good ones to choose from.

Start with one "good nutrition" day a week and five or ten minutes of walking a day. Gradually increase your "good nutrition" days and your minutes of exercise. Never decrease your good habits even when you cannot give up bad ones.

Some bad habits are a result of genetics, or a lifetime of inactivity or wrong environmental surroundings. Whatever the cause, you may need to make a major change in your lifestyle. The people who do this best are those who do it on their own without therapy.

Addictions or habits can also be caused by the pharmacological addictive properties of certain drugs like alcohol, caffeine, or nicotine, of chemicals (including sugar) in junk foods, or by a person's social situation, attitudes and expectations. Almost everyone can control their habits and addictions if they **believe** that they can. Only you can quit your habit; nobody can quit for you.

Creating a healthier body for ourselves enables us to enjoy our lives more fully. The healthier your body is, the easier it will be to refrain from bad habits. Using exercise, nutrition, breathing techniques and relaxation, you will begin to build self-confidence, enable easy withdrawal from a habit and provide alternatives that can be more satisfying than the habit itself.

Sometimes changing a habit may involve several attempts and methods to change. If one doesn't help, another may. The important thing is to retain your awareness of what you want to change for yourself, accept yourself regardless of how slow or fast you change, and try again. As you continue to move toward what you want for yourself, the habit will fall away.

The most powerful motivation for changing a habit is the determination that "I want to improve the quality of my life. I want greater health and vitality. I want to increase my capacity to enjoy living." To change a habit, we must base our efforts on the desire to live a higher quality life.

MOTIVATION

The difference between those who are successful at changing habits, lifestyle and other aspects of their life and those who fail is the degree of motivation. You may have been telling yourself for years that you want to lose weight and get in shape, or quit smoking or get a new job. But getting out and doing something about it depends on just how important these things are to you and how they make you feel. You have to feel an urge to want to do something and know **why** you want to change something. You have to decide to do it **now**. With enough motivation you don't even need to think about having will power — it comes naturally. Next, find someone who can help you or lead you in the right direction so you can help yourself.

Following is a five point plan to help you get started on a motivational path to good health:

(1.) Set easy, short-term goals and list the steps it will take to achieve them. Know exactly what it is you want and how to go about doing it — the right way. Find someone who can give you advice, or visit your library or book store. Take your time. Change an aspect of your lifestyle gradually, with patience and a positive frame of mind.

(2.) Find a person or group of people who can help keep you going. "Support is essential to keep a lot of people going," says Susan Smith Jones, who holds a Ph.D. in health sciences and operates the consulting firm **Health Unlimited**, in Los Angeles, California.

(3.) Experiment for a month or two until you find the program that most appropriately suits you. Give yourself time to adjust.

"Behavioral scientists say that it takes the body 21 days to accept new behavior," says Dr. Jones. "If you give up sugar, for instance, you must keep at it for at least 21 days before your body accepts the change as natural. Set goals that are so realistic and easy to achieve that you won't fail. Take it one day at a time."

Also, remember that the first group, doctor or program that you find may not be what you want or what you need. But don't be discouraged and stop. Keep on looking. Eventually you'll find a way toward your goals that you enjoy and that work.

To be healthy you must believe in good health, what it means and how you will benefit from it. Most of us are brought up worrying about how to be ready for illness or disease as opposed to learning what optimal health really is.

(4.) Be flexible — leave a little room for error. No exercise or diet program should be so rigid that it doesn't leave room for a little diversion.

Rigid programs are just simply too difficult to follow. A day off from exercise or an occasional dip of ice cream are all part of handling a practical long-term program.

(5.) Visualize how good the "new you" will look and feel.

Actually seeing the physical results is the best way to keep your motivation in high gear. When you feel healthy and are in shape, you'll also feel happy, and as Dr. Jones states, "You'll begin to celebrate life!"

Susan Smith Jones shares her fresh, dynamic approach to life and to developing your fullest potential through her book *THE MAIN INGREDIENTS: Positive Thinking, Exercise, and Diet* and her new series of cassette tapes called appropriately, **CELEBRATE LIFE.**

GOOD HEALTH CAN COST LESS

The average American spends over $1000 per year seeing doctors, staying in hospitals, and purchasing drugs and over the counter medicines. This does not even take into account less obvious costs: loss of earnings, family disruption and emotional and general hardships suffered by family members. Even if you have medical insurance, you are still paying for sickness and medical costs through increases in insurance rates. Six of the ten leading causes of death in the United States are directly attributable to our lifestyle, diet, exercise and the way we cope with stress.

Regular exercise, a positive mental attitude, and a daily concern for good nutrition will put you on the road toward good health and feeling better.

Contrary to popular belief, eating healthy foods can actually be more economical than the typical American diet.

Eating more complex carbohydrate foods like whole grains, beans, peas, vegetables and fruits, and less of the more expensive meat and dairy foods, refined, processed and packaged foods and foods high in sugar and oils can result in a substantial savings in your food budget. Just as you wouldn't think of purchasing a cheap piece of furniture that could fall apart after a few uses, neither should you think of buying cheap food that causes your body to fall apart. When you buy food, remember that good health at any price is priceless!

If you have your own garden and do more of your own cooking, you can not only save money but you can be eating fresher ingredients and avoiding overcooked packaged foods, additives, excess salt, sugar and fat.

Choosing and preparing foods in such a way that you preserve their vital nutrients can be a joy, because you know that you are nourishing your body's physical as well as mental health. It's fun too!

THE RESPONSIBILITY IS YOURS

We cannot make you healthy, only you can do that. It is important that **you** assume the responsibility of attaining total health. Good health is not a matter of luck or fate. You have to work at it.

You can achieve a higher level of wellness through the acquiring of knowledge, growth in personal awareness, positive changes in your outlook on life and changes in your lifestyle. It is not as difficult as many people think. Along with good nutrition and exercise, these steps toward health and wellness include certain attitudes and practices that enhance your health and enrich your life. By using them, you can feel good, have abundant energy, vibrant optimal well-being and participate more fully in a longer life.

Your future depends on you. Only you can change its outcome by becoming aware of, and making the proper choices toward, the most healthful existence possible.

The first thing you must do is to make the decision to start now and to make the commitment to take responsibility for your own body and your own health.

You must **believe** that you can and do have the ability to follow the "Laws of Health". Most of all, **do not give up** trying to attain good health. Always be positive. Put yourself in command of your willpower and outside influences. Decide what changes you want to make for improvement. Choose an aspect of your nutritional habits or of your lifestyle that you feel you can successfully change most easily.

Set some goals for yourself and develop a plan that you can follow. Pay close attention to how you feel at all times so you know that the changes you are making are indeed making you feel better. You can then eliminate unhealthful aspects of your lifestyle and concentrate on increasing healthful ways of living.

Other things you can do to help are to change your environment, if possible. Look for people and social systems that are compatible and supportive of your desired behavior.

Focus on the positive effects rather than on what you are losing as a result of the change. Never decrease your good habits even when you cannot give up your bad ones.

Learn through observing others — healthy others, especially those with whom you can easily identify.

When in doubt, consult with those who have knowledge on specific areas that may be helpful to you.

Learn from your failures. Behavior changes take time. Thomas Edison was once asked why he persisted in his desire to invent a new type of battery in the face of frequent failure. He replied, "What failure? I have no failures. Now I know 50,000 ways it won't work." You are not a failure when you fail.

You now have the information you need to live a long and healthy life. All you need to do is to put it into practice and you will enjoy each and every day of your life even more.

It feels so good to be healthy that change comes much easier than you think.

By implementing a new HEALTHSTYLE gradually, you will enjoy every new experience. Soon they will be a natural part of each and every day of your life.

With a little inspiration, motivation and know-how, you can easily begin to undertake a lifelong program of wellness.

Take charge of your life, improve your diet and your attitude, begin a good exercise program and replace stressful worry with a positive plan.

"Each individual has responsibility to the self, to ensure that he or she remains physically, mentally and spiritually fit and healthy throughout life."

Charles L. Pelton, M.D. (author of "Doctor, My Bill Is Too High")

WHERE TO FIND NUTRITIONAL PRODUCTS AND INFORMATION

Many products mentioned in this book are not available in regular supermarkets or drug stores. Most good health and natural food stores carry the majority of the products mentioned, as well as many other healthful products.

These stores carry a large variety of whole grain products ranging from bread to cake mixes. You will be able to find many familiar-looking foods without excess salt, sugar, fats, and chemical additives, as well as a good selection of books on special health topics and some of the most natural body care items available. Remember that you should nourish your skin with as much concern as you do the rest of your body.

Never be afraid to ask for a product that you can't find. It can usually be ordered for you if the store does not carry it on its shelves. Health and natural food stores exist to offer you products and services that will keep you healthy. Most good stores have one or more nutrition consultants on their staff who are always willing to help with any questions you may have.

Healthful foods can even be found in abundance in your local supermarket — although they may be upstaged by flashily packaged processed foods that are more profitable for your supermarket. You may not notice them, but they're there. Brown rice and other whole grains, all types of beans, raw nuts and seeds, fresh fruits and vegetables, unprocessed cheeses, lean meat and chicken, fish and low-fat dairy products — all these are natural, whole, healthful foods.

Remember: healthful foods are those consumed in as close to their original form as possible — not battered, coated, precooked, or made "convenient" in some other way. Try to get the organically-grown versions of these foods as often as possible.

OTHER RESOURCES TO HELP YOU

In addition to personal actions you can take on your own, there are community programs, groups, organizations and businesses that can assist you and your family to make the changes you want to make. There are many sources of information you can use to stay healthy and to start a new HEALTHSTYLE.

Some of these sources are:

1. YMCA and YWCA
2. Health and Natural Food Stores
3. Nutrition and preventive minded doctors of all types
4. American Heart Association
5. American Cancer Society
6. Other such Health Organizations
7. Stress Reduction Clinics
8. Weight Control Clinics
9. Health and Fitness Clubs
10. County Health Department
11. Alcohol and Drug Abuse Organizations
12. Vo-Tech or other community college classes
13. County Extension Service

To help you locate preventive and nutrition minded health professionals in your area we are providing three addresses to which you can write for national directories of these practitioners. They include doctors, osteopaths, chiropractors, dentists, naturopaths and other alternative health specialists.

International Academy of Preventive Medicine
10950 Grandview, Suite 469
34 Corporate Woods
Overland Park, Kansas 66210
(913) 684-8720

American Holistic Medical Association
6932 Little River Turnpike
Annandale, Virginia 22003
(703) 642-5880

Medical Services Department
Alacer Corporation
Box 6180
Buena Park, California 90622

There are also many holistic and nutrition/natural healing clinics and hospitals around the country which stress disease **prevention,** as well as drugless, non-invasive healing methods, resorting to drugs and surgery only when absolutely necessary. Many of these emphasize **wellness** — that state of harmony between body and mind, emotions and spirit.

Part of your self-responsibility should be to establish a 'client' relationship with your physician or other health-care professional rather than maintaining a 'patient' relationship. Regarding yourself as a client, you and your doctor should then discuss such things as side effects of drugs and possible alternatives to taking medication or undergoing surgery. If you have a health problem that is stress or diet related, you and your doctor should discuss natural ways to correct your problem. If your doctor prefers to treat you as a patient rather than as a client, you should find another.

You should also ask your doctor if he is familiar with nutritional approaches to better health. If not, perhaps you may want to change doctors. Doctors with degrees of D.O., M.D., D.C., N.D., or D.D.S. may be able to help you. You may wish to ask your doctor if he belongs to any professional preventive, nutritional or holistic medical associations.

"The doctor of the future will give no medicine, but rather will interest his patients in the care of the human frame, in diet, and in the cause and prevention of disease."   Thomas Edison

CHIROPRACTIC

Because many people are confused about the medical field of Chiropractic, and because we feel it offers specific benefits for many health problems, we decided to have Dr. Kenneth Luedtke, D.C., President of the American Chiropractic Association give us the following brief explanation of the benefits and treatment methods of Chiropractic:

Chiropractic is a branch of the healing arts which is concerned with human health and disease processes. Doctors of chiropractic are doctors who give special attention to spinal mechanics, musculoskeletal, neurological, vascular and nutritional relationships.

Chiropractic is built upon three related scientific theories and principles:

1. Disease May Be Caused by Disturbances of the Nervous System. Conditions which irritate the nervous system, and to which the body cannot successfully adapt, produce abnormal changes in the pattern of nerve impulses. Thus many functional disturbances are triggered which, if unchecked, lead to disease processes.

2. Disturbances of the Nervous System May Be Caused by Derangements of the Musculoskeletal Structure. Extended abnormal involvement of the nervous system may result from disturbances, strains and stresses arising within the musculoskeletal system due to man's attempt to maintain erect posture.

3. Disturbances of the Nervous System May Cause or Aggravate Disease in Various Parts or Functions of the Body. Almost any component of the nervous system may directly or indirectly cause reactions within any other component by means of reflex mediation.

The doctor of chiropractic conducts a systematic and thorough physical examination using the methods, techniques and instruments that are standard with all health professions. In addition, a postural and spinal analysis is included.

Chiropractic treatment methods are determined by the scope of practice authorized by state law. In all areas, however, these methods do not include the use of prescription drugs or surgery. Chiropractic is a drug-free, nonsurgical science. Essentially, treatment methods include the chiropractic adjustment, necessary dietary advice and nutritional supplementation, physiotherapeutic measures, professional counsel and whatever other procedure is necessary for the best health care of the patient's complaint.

The chiropractic corrective adjustment is made only after careful analysis, delivered in a specific manner, to achieve a predetermined goal. It is a precise, delicate maneuver, requiring special bio-engineering skills and a deftness not unlike that required for a surgeon. Rarely is the process painful.

Most chiropractic corrective adjustments are made upon the joints, especially those of the spinal column. Some techniques, however, are light-touch reflex adjustments which involve the neurovascular, neurolymphatic and neuromuscular systems — similar to the systems involved in Chinese meridian therapy. These surface techniques are far more than massage or trigger-point releases, for they must involve careful diagnosis and be scientifically applied after comprehensive chiropractic training.

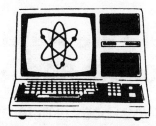

COMPUTERIZED PROGRAMS TO ASSIST YOU IN YOUR QUEST FOR TOTAL HEALTH

To help you take that important first step in assessing your current level of health and wellness, AMERICAN HEALTH AND NUTRITION offers two valuable and beneficial computerized health promotion programs. Dr. Leslie Salov, Director of the Vision and Health Center in Wisconsin and Medical Advisor to AMERICAN HEALTH AND NUTRITION states, "These programs will give people in-depth information about the many factors affecting their personal health, and are very helpful in directing them toward improving their well-being and achieving total health."

Your Body Is Different Than Anybody Else's

Don't Guess About Your Vitamin and Mineral Needs!

If you are confused about your vitamin and mineral needs, you can get a personalized program which evaluates the balance and metabolism of **your** body. The **Comprehensive Health & Nutrition Profile**© (Personal Health and Nutrition Assessment) is a scientific computerized read-out taken from data relating to you, **your** eating habits, **your** lifestyle and **your** body's needs.

It utilizes the latest developments in computer hardware and software to give you an accurate analysis of your nutritional health.

The report provides a **Comprehensive Health and Nutrition Profile**© with a step-by-step plan to fine-tune your body and program your energy. It will show you what you need and don't need in nutrition to gain optimum personal metabolic balance. What you need in calories, in protein, fats, fiber and carbohydrates. What you need in vitamins and minerals. What you need in wholesome natural foods.

You can save time, save money, save confusion and save your future by knowing what **your** body really needs. This health evaluation is available from Amerian Health and Nutrition for $19.95. Or a free brochure is available upon request.

Now there are ways for you to live longer and happier!

Recognize that your body is different from others. Find out what it takes to keep it running efficiently.

People nowadays are more concerned about their health and life expectancy. And that's good. Except, most people think that exercising or keeping their weight down is the total answer. They are grossly wrong.

The body is a complex mechanism and every person is different. What is right for one person may be totally wrong for the other — possibly even harmful to that person's health.

Possibly you know everything about yourself, but have the relationships of your family health history, environment and habits been put into a meaningful picture? Has a measure and analysis been made so as to provide you with a Comprehensive Health Profile? Probably not!

Has the statistical information on *you* been fed into a computer: your life style inventory, your laboratory tests, your physical measurements, your biographical data, your family and personal health histories, your medication history, your physical activity profile, your drinking status and problem drinking inventory, your smoking status and history, your stress inventory, your relaxation, your safety and occupation survey, your nutrition and eating habits analysis?

WHAT DOES THE COMPREHENSIVE LIFE EXTENSION PROFILE© CONTAIN?

Data from specific health tests is incorporated as is all the information from other surveys; height and weight

Comprehensive Life Extension Profile™

measurements; skinfold test for determining percent body fat; heart rate and blood pressure; lung function tests and eating habits. From this data the computer generates:

- Your Comprehensive Risk Profile (covering more than 20 major risk factors).
- Your Health Hazard Appraisal (listing your personal quotient for consideration against the 10-12 leading causes of death.)
- Your Health Age and Longevity Appraisal.
- Your Nutrition Profile: An analysis of calorie, protein, fat, fiber and carbohydrate intake.
- Your Fitness Profile: Provides ideal weight and exercise recommendations, heart and lung capacity values, and the average number of calories you are using per day.

All reports include personalized recommendations for reducing risk and enhancing health.

This Comprehensive Life Extension Profile™ is available from American Health and Nutrition for $19.95. A free brochure is available.

DESIDERATA

Go placidly amid the noise and haste, and remember what peace there may be in silence. As far as possible without surrender, be on good terms with all persons.

Speak your truths quietly and clearly; and listen to others, even the dull and ignorant; they too have their story. Avoid loud and aggressive persons, they are vexations to the spirit.

If you compare yourself with others, you may become vain and bitter; for always there will be greater and lesser persons than yourself. Enjoy your achievements as well as your plans.

Keep interested in your own career, however humble; it is a real possession in the changing fortunes of time.

Exercise caution in your business affairs; for the world is full of trickery. But let this not blind you to what virtue there is; many persons strive for high ideals and everywhere life is full of heroism.

Be yourself. Especially, do not feign affection. Neither be cynical about love; for in the face of all aridity and disenchantment it is perennial as the grass.

Take kindly the counsel of the years, gracefully surrendering the things of youth. Nurture strength of spirit to shield you in misfortune. But do not distress yourself with imaginings. Many fears are born of fatigue and loneliness.

Beyond a wholesome discipline, be gentle with yourself. You are a child of the universe, no less than the trees and the stars; you have a right to be here.

And whether or not it is clear to you, no doubt the universe is unfolding as it should.

Therefore be at peace with God, whatever you conceive Him to be, and whatever your labors and aspirations, in the noisy confusion of life, keep peace with your soul.

With all its shame, drudgery, and broken dreams, it is still a beautiful world. Be careful. Strive to be happy.

by Max Ehrmann

SELECTED LIST OF BOOKS AND TAPES TO HELP YOU ON YOUR WAY TO A NEW HEALTHSTYLE

Along with our own experience, we have researched many publications in compiling information for this book. So many of them agree on certain topics that we felt it was not necessary to include a lot of footnotes and references. However, we are providing the following partial list of books and tapes that have been helpful to us and that we highly recommend to you for further information on a specific topic that may be of interest to you. These books and tapes are easy to read and understand and can make positive contributions to you in learning more about TOTAL HEALTH and WELLNESS. For a brief summary of these and other publications, please write to us at:

Health and Fitness Information
American Health and Nutrition
7 N. Pinckney, Suite 225
Madison, WI 53703

We'll also be happy to give you more information on how you can obtain some of the products we've mentioned in this book.

Books:
Aerobics for Women by Ken and Mildred Cooper
Cancer and Its Nutritional Therapies by Dr. Richard Passwater
Complete Meditation by Steven Kravette
Complete Relaxation by Steven Kravette
The Complete Shopper's Guide to Health and Natural Food Stores by Christopher Kilham, N.D.
Creative Visualization by S. Gawain
Deaf Smith Country Cookbook by Marjorie Winnford, Susan Hillyard and Mary Faulk Koock
Encyclopedia of Common Diseases by *Prevention Magazine*
Every Woman's Book by Paavo Airola, N.D., Ph.D.
Feed Your Kids Right by Dr. Lendon Smith
Feed Yourself Right by Dr. Lendon Smith
Feeling Great by Jeanne Segal, Ph.D.
Fit or Fat? by Covert Bailey
For the Love of Food "The Complete Natural Foods Cookbook" by Jeanne Martin
Fourteen Days to a Wellness Lifestyle: The Easy, Effective, and Fun Way to Optimum Health by Donald Ardell
Freedom From Stress-Holistic Approach by Phillip Neurenberger, Ph.D.
Get A Job in 60 Seconds by Steven Kravette
Goodbye Blues (Breaking the Tranquilizer Habit the Natural Way) by Bernard Green, Ph.D.
Guide to Stress Reduction by L. John Mason, Ph.D.
Happiness is Now by Amrit Desai
Heartsong Tofu Cookbook by Joani and Bob Heartsong
How To Be A Couple and Still Be Free by Tina Tessina, M.A. and Riley Smith, M.A.
How to Eat Without Meat by Judi and Shari Zucker

How to Feel Younger Longer by Jane Kinderlehrer
How to Keep Your Family Fit and Healthy by Bonnie Prudden
How to Talk So Kids Will Listen and How to Listen So Kids Will Talk by Adelle Faber and Elaine Mazlish
Human Life Styling (Keeping Whole in the 20th Century) by John McCamy and James Presley
Inner Balance by Eliot Goldwag
Jane Brody's Nutrition Book
Jogging by William Bowerman and W. E. Harris, M.D.
Joy of Quitting by Burton and Wohl
Kicking the Coffee Habit by Charles Wetherall
Kinship For All Life by J. Allen Boone
Know Your Nutrition by Linda Clark
Laurel's Kitchen by L. Robertson, C. Flinders and B. Godfrey
Lifeplan for Health and Fitness by Dennis and David Singsank
Maggie's Womans Book by Maggie Lettvin
Man's Body: An Owner's Manual by The Diagram Group
Natural Sleep (How To Get Your Share) by Phillip Goldberg and Daniel Kaufman
Nerve Force (Building Powerful Nerve Energy) by Paul and Patricia Bragg, N.D., Ph.D.
Never Say Diet Book by Richard Simmons
Nutrition Almanac by Nutrition Search Inc.
Nutrition and Vitamin Therapy by Michael Lesser, M.D.
Nutritional Approach to Super Health by Kurt Donsbach, Ph.D.
Ourselves, Our Children by Boston Women's Collective
Parent Book by Harold Bressler, Jr. and Thomas P. Kelley
People's Pharmacy-2 by Joe Graedon
Practical Encyclopedia of Natural Healing by Mark Bricklin of Prevention Magazine
Pritikin Permanent Weight Loss Manual by Nathan Pritikin
Pritikin Program for Diet and Exercise by Nathan Pritikin with Patrick M. McGrady, Jr.
The Prevention of Alcoholism through Nutrition by Dr. Roger J. Williams
Rebounding Aerobics by Morton Walker, D.P.M. and Frank Angelo
Recipes for a Small Planet by Ellen Buchman Ewald
Rodale's Encyclopedia of Natural Home Remedies by Mark Bricklin
Self Assertion for Women by Pamela Butler
Sigh of Relief (The First Aid Handbook for Childhood Emergencies) by Martin Green
Starting Small in the Wilderness: Family Guide to the Outdoors by N. Doan of the Sierra Club
Stretching by Bob Anderson
Success Through a Positive Mental Attitude by Napoleon Hill and W. Clement Stone
Sugar Blues by William Dufty and Gloria Swanson
Talking Together by Sherod Miller, Elam Nunally and Daniel Wackman
Vitamin Bible by Earl Mindell
Women and the Crisis in Sex Hormones by Barbara Seamans and Gideon Seamans, M.D.
You Are Greater Than You Know by Lou Austin
Your Personal Vitamin Profile by Dr. Michael Colgan
Your Second Life (Vitality and Growth in Middle or Later Years) by Gay Gail Luce
Tapes:
Building Health Immunity by Dr. Kurt Donsbach
Choosing A Food Supplement by Dr. Kurt Donsbach
Easing Into Sleep by Dr. Emmett Miller
The Healing Journey by Dr. Emmett Miller
Health and Success: The Winning Pair by A. Karlins
Health and Wellness by Dr. Emmett Miller
High Blood Pressure (And Low Blood Pressure) by Dr. Kurt Donsbach
How to Live 365 Days a Year by Dr. John Schindler
How To Live With Another Person by Dr. John Viscott

Imagine Yourself Slim: Transforming Your Self Image, Attitudes and Behavior by Dr. Emmett Miller

Letting Go of Stress by Dr. Emmett Miller

The Main Ingredients: Positive Thinking, Exercise and Nutrition by Susan Smith Jones, Ph.D.

Relaxing Techniques for Reducing Stress by AMERICAN HEALTH AND NUTRITION

Other Valuable Health Resources:

- TV: Cable Health Network
- Magazines: American Health, Prevention and many others available in book stores, health food stores, supermarkets and drug stores.
- Consumer Health Organizations: Natural Food Associates, National Health Federation, Center for Science in the Public Interest, People's Medical Society (Emmaus, PA) and many others.

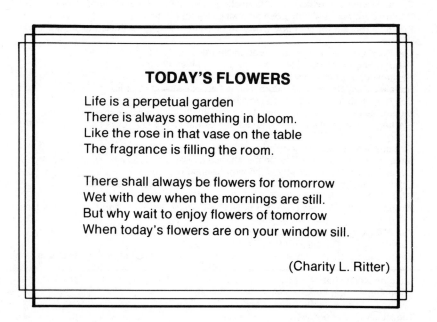

TODAY'S FLOWERS

Life is a perpetual garden
There is always something in bloom.
Like the rose in that vase on the table
The fragrance is filling the room.

There shall always be flowers for tomorrow
Wet with dew when the mornings are still.
But why wait to enjoy flowers of tomorrow
When today's flowers are on your window sill.

(Charity L. Ritter)

COMPOSITION OF FOODS
100 grams, edible portion (3.6 oz.)

(dash (—) denotes lack of reliable data for a constituent believed to be present in measurable amount)

This is only a partial listing for you to use as a guide in learning the nutritional content of other foods.

FOOD	CALORIES	PROTEINS grams	FATS grams	CARBOHYDRATES grams	CALCIUM mg.	PHOSPHORUS mg.	MAGNESIUM mg.	IRON mg.	SODIUM mg.	POTASSIUM mg.	VITAMIN A VALUE IU	B1 mg.	B2 mg.	NIACIN mg.	VITAMIN C mg.
ALMONDS, raw	598	18.6	54.2	19.5	234	504	270	4.7	4.0	773	0	.24	.92	3.5	trace
APPLES	58	.2	.6	14.5	7	10	8	.3	1	110	90	.03	.02	.4	7-20
APPLE JUICE, canned or bottled	47	.1	trace	11.9	6	9	4	.6	1	101	—	.01	.02	.1	1.0
APRICOTS, raw	51	1.0	.2	1.8	17	23	12	.5	1	281	2,700	0.3	.04	.6	10
ASPARAGUS, raw spears	26	2.5	.2	5.0	22	62	20	1.0	2	278	900	.18	.20	1.5	33
AVOCADOS	167	2.1	16.4	6.3	10	42	45	.6	4	604	290	.11	.20	1.6	14
BANANAS	85	1.1	.2	22.2	8	26	33	.7	1	370	190	.05	.06	.7	10
BARLEY, pearled	349	8.2	1.0	78.8	16	189	37	2.0	3	160	0	.12	.05	3.1	0
BEANS, white, cooked	118	7.8	.6	21.2	50	148	37	2.7	7	416	0	.14	.07	.7	0
red, cooked	347	7.8	.5	21.4	38	140	—	2.7	3	340	trace	.11	.06	.7	—
pinto, raw	349	22.9	1.2	63.7	135	457	—	6.4	10	984	—	.84	.21	2.2	—
lima, cooked	138	8.2	.6	25.6	29	154	48	3.1	2	612	—	.13	.06	.7	—
mung, sprouted, raw	38	3.8	.2	6.6	19	64	—	1.3	5	223	20	.13	.13	.8	19
green, raw	32	1.9	.2	7.1	56	44	32	.8	7	243	600	.8	.11	.5	19
BEEF POT ROAST	291	27.4	19	0	11.9	—	—	3.4	—	—	35.7	.05	.21	4.2	—
fat trimmed	200	31.4	7.1	0	14.3	—	—	3.8	—	—	14.3	.06	.23	4.7	—
BEETS, red, cooked	32	1.1	.1	7.2	14	23	15	.5	43	208	20	.03	.04	.3	6
BLUEBERRIES, raw	62	.7	.5	15.3	15	13	6	1.0	1	81	100	.03	.06	.4	14
BRAZIL NUTS, raw	654	14.3	66.9	10.9	186	693	225	3.4	1	715	trace	.96	.12	1.6	—
BROCCOLI, raw spears	32	3.6	.3	5.9	103	78	24	1.1	15	382	2,500	.10	.23	.9	113
BUCKWHEAT, whole grain	335	11.7	2.4	72.9	114	282	229	3.1	—	448	0	.60	—	4.4	0

	CALORIES	PROTEINS grams	FATS grams	CARBOHYDRATES grams	CALCIUM mg.	PHOSPHORUS mg.	MAGNESIUM mg.	IRON mg.	SODIUM mg.	POTASSIUM mg.	VITAMIN A VALUE IU	B1 mg.	B2 mg.	NIACIN mg.	VITAMIN C mg.
BUTTER, salted	716	.6	81	.4	20	16	2	0	987	23	3,300				0
CABBAGE, raw	24	1.3	.2	5.4	49	29	13	.4	20	233	130	.05	.05	.3	47
red, raw	31	2.0	.2	6.9	42	35		.8	26	268	40	.09	.06	.4	61
CAROB FLOUR	180	4.5	1.4	80.7	352	81	23								
CARROTS, raw	42	1.1	.2	9.7	37	36	23	.7	47	341	11,000	.06	.05	.6	8
CASHEW NUTS	561	17.2	45.7	29.3	38	373	267	3.8	15	464	100	.43	.25	1.8	
CAULIFLOWER, raw	27	2.7	.2	5.2	25	56	24	1.1	13	295	60	.11	.10	.7	78
CELERY, raw	17	.9	.1	3.9	39	28	22	.3	126	341	240	.03	.03	.3	9
CHARD, Swiss, raw	25	2.4	.3	4.6	88	39	65	3.2	147	550	6,500	.06	.17	.5	32
CHEESE, Cheddar	398	25.0	32.2	2.1	750	478	45	1.0	700	82	1,310	.03	.46	.1	
Cottage, uncreamed	86	17.0	.3	2.7	90	175		.4	290	72	10	.03	.28	.1	
Swiss	370	27.5	28.0	1.7	925	563		.9	710	104	1140	.01	.40	.1	
CHICKEN, broiled, without skin	136.8	36	3.6	0	11.9			1.75			95	.06	.22	14	
fried, with skin	205	33	6.6	1.3	9.5			1.6			95	.05	.19	9	
COCONUT, dried	662	7.2	64.9	23.0	26	187	90	3.3	trace	588	0	.06	.04	.6	0
CORN SWEET, cooked on the cob	91	3.3	1.0	21.0	3	89	19	.6	6	196	400	.12	.10	1.4	9
CUCUMBERS, raw	15	.9	.1	3.4	25	27	11	1.1	1	160	250	.03	.04	.2	11
DATES	274	2.2	.5	72.9	59	63	58	3.0		648		.09	.10	2.2	0
EGGS, cooked, whole	163	12.9	11.5	.9	54	205		2.3	122	129	1,180	.09	.28	.1	0
FIGS, dried	274	4.3	1.3	69.1	126	77	71	3.0	34	640	80	.10	.10	.7	
FILBERTS (hazelnuts)	634	12.6	62.4	16.7	209	337	84	3.4	2	704		.46		.0	
FISH, Flounder or Cod, baked or broiled	81	19.54		0	38			1.3				.04	.07	3	
fried	232	18	13	8	33			1.3	1			.09	.1	1.8	
GRAPEFRUIT	41	.5	.1	10.6	16	16	12	.4	1	135	80	.04	.02	.2	38

	CALORIES	PROTEINS grams	FATS grams	CARBOHYDRATES grams	CALCIUM	PHOSPHORUS mg	MAGNESIUM mg	IRON mg	SODIUM mg	POTASSIUM mg	VITAMIN A VALUE IU	B1 mg	B2 mg	NIACIN mg	VITAMIN C mg
GRAPES	69	1.3	1.0	15.7	16	12	13	.4	3	158	100	.05	.03	.3	4
HONEY	304	.3	0	82.3	5	6	3	.5	5	51	0	trace	.04	.3	1
KALE, leaves, raw	53	6.0	.8	9.0	249	93	37	2.7	75	378	10,000	.17	.26	2.1	186
•LENTILS, dry, cooked	106	7.8	trace	19.3	25	119	80	2.1	—	249	20	.07	.06	.6	0
LETTUCE, raw, Romaine	18	1.3	.3	3.5	68	25	11	1.4	9	264	1,900	.05	.08	.4	18
Iceberg, New York	13	.9	.1	2.9	20	22	13	.5	9	175	330	.06	.06	.3	6
MILK, cow's, whole	65	3.5	3.5	4.9	118	93	13	trace	50	144	140	.03	.17	.1	1
skim	36	3.6	.1	5.1	121	95	14	trace	52	145	trace	.04	.18	.1	1
dry, skim non-instant	363	35.9	.8	52.3	1,308	1,016	143	.6	532	1,745	30	.35	1.80	.9	7
MILK, goat's, raw	67	3.2	4.0	4.6	129	106	17	.1	34	180	160	.04	.11	.3	1
MILLET, whole-grain	327	9.9	2.9	72.9	20	311	162	6.8	—	430	0	.73	.38	2.3	0
MUSHROOMS, raw	28	2.7	.3	4.4	6	116	13	.8	15	414	trace	.10	.46	4.2	3
MUSKMELONS, raw, cantaloupe	30	.7	.1	7.5	14	16	16	.4	12	251	3,400	.04	.03	.6	33
OATMEAL or rolled oats, cooked	55	2.0	1.0	9.7	9	57	21	.6	—	61	0	.08	.02	.1	0
ORANGES	49	1.0	.2	12.2	41	20	11	.4	1	200	200	.10	.04	.4	50
ORANGE JUICE, raw	45	.7	.2	10.2	11	17	11	.2	1	200	200	.09	.03	.4	50
PEACHES	38	.6	.1	9.7	9	19	10	.5	1	202	1,330	.02	.05	1.0	7
PEANUTS, raw, with skins	564	26.0	47.5	18.6	69	401	206	2.1	5	674	—	1.14	.13	17.2	0
PEARS	61	.7	.4	15.3	8	11	7	.3	2	130	20	.02	.04	.1	4
PEAS, green, cooked	71	5.4	.4	12.1	23	89	—	1.8	1	196	540	.28	.11	2.3	20
split, cooked	115	8.0	.3	20.8	11	89	—	1.7	13	296	40	.15	.09	.9	—
PECANS	687	9.2	71.2	14.6	73	289	142	2.4	trace	603	130	.86	.13	.9	—
PEPPERS, raw, sweet, green	22	1.2	.2	4.8	9	22	18	trace	13	213	420	.08	.08	.5	128
PINEAPPLE	52	0.4	0.2	13.7	17	8	13	.7	1	146	70	.09	.03	.2	17
PLUMS	75	.8	.2	19.7	12	18	9	0.5	1	170	300	.03	.03	.5	4
POTATOES, raw	76	2.1	.1	17.1	7	53	34	.6	3	407	trace	.10	.04	1.5	20

	CALORIES	PROTEINS grams	FATS grams	CARBOHYDRATES grams	CALCIUM	PHOSPHORUS mg.	MAGNESIUM mg.	IRON mg.	SODIUM mg.	POTASSIUM mg.	VITAMIN A VALUE IU	B1 mg.	B2 mg.	NIACIN mg.	VITAMIN C mg.
baked in skin	93	2.6	.1	21.1	9	65	—	.7	4	503	trace	.10	.04	1.7	20
PUMPKIN SEEDS, raw	553	29.0	46.7	15.0	51	1,144	—	11.2	—	—	70	.24	.19	2.4	—
RAISINS, natural	289	2.5	.2	77.4	62	101	35	3.5	27	763	20	.11	.08	.5	1
RASPBERRIES, red	57	1.2	.5	13.6	22	22	20	0.9	1	168	130	.03	.09	0.9	25
RICE, brown, cooked	119	2.5	.6	25.5	12	73	29	.5	3	70	0	.09	.02	1.4	0
RYE, whole-grain	334	12.1	1.7	73.4	38	376	115	3.7	1	467	0	.43	.22	1.6	0
SESAME SEEDS, dry, whole	563	18.6	49.1	21.6	1,160	616	181	10.5	60	725	30	.98	.24	5.4	0
SOYBEANS, dry, raw	403	34.1	17.7	33.5	226	554	265	8.4	5	1,677	80	1.10	.31	2.2	—
cooked	130	11.0	5.7	10.8	73	179	—	2.7	2	540	30	.21	.09	.6	0
SOYBEAN CURD (TOFU)	72	7.8	4.2	2.4	128	126	111	1.9	7	42	0	.06	.03	.1	—
SOYBEAN MILK, powder	429	41.8	20.03	28.0	278	—	300	—	—	—	—	—	—	—	—
SPINACH, raw	26	3.2	.3	4.3	93	51	88	3.1	71	470	8,100	.10	.20	.6	51
SQUASH, winter, cooked (baked)	63	1.8	.4	15.4	28	48	17	.8	1	461	4,200	.05	.13	.7	13
STRAWBERRIES	37	.7	.5	8.4	21	21	12	1.0	1	164	60	.03	.07	.6	59
SUNFLOWER SEED KERNELS, raw	560	24.0	47.3	19.9	120	837	38	7.1	30	920	50	1.96	.23	5.4	—
TOMATOES, ripe, raw	22	1.1	.2	4.7	13	27	14	.5	3	244	900	.06	.04	.7	23
WALNUTS, English	651	14.8	64.0	15.8	99	380	131	3.1	2	450	30	.33	.13	.9	2
WATERMELON	26	.5	.2	6.4	7	10	8	.5	1	100	590	.03	.03	.2	7
WHEAT, whole grain, winter	330	12.3	1.8	71.7	46	354	160	3.4	3	370	—	.52	.12	4.3	0
WHEAT BRAN	213	16.0	4.6	61.9	119	1,276	490	14.9	9	1,121	0	.72	.35	21.0	0
WHEAT GERM, raw	363	26.6	10.9	46.7	72	1,118	336	9.4	3	827	0	2.01	.68	4.2	0
YEAST, brewer's debittered	283	38.8	1.0	38.4	210	1,753	231	17.3	121	1,894	trace	15.61	4.28	37.9	trace
YOGURT, from whole milk	62	3.0	3.4	4.9	111	87	12	trace	47	132	140	.03	.16	.1	1
from skimmed milk	50	3.4	1.7	5.2	120	94	13	trace	51	143	70	.04	.18	.1	1

SOURCES: Agriculture Handbook No. 8., U.S. Dept. Agric. Washington D.C., Home and Garden Bulletin No. 72.

INDEX

NOTES

If you have enjoyed reading this book and would like to share it with others, please consider giving it as a gift. For anyone who wishes an extra copy **just cut and mail** one of the forms below.

If you know of any organization or business that might like to offer LIFE-PLAN FOR HEALTH AND FITNESS to their employees, members, customers, clients, etc. please let us know and we will be happy to provide purchasing information for larger orders. We would also be happy to send information to any organization interested in offering LIFEPLAN FOR HEALTH AND FITNESS in their fund-raising programs.

If you wish to receive a copy of LIFEPLAN FOR HEALTH AND FITNESS, fill out and mail this card.

Please send to the following address:

NAME _____

ADDRESS _____

CITY _____

STATE _____ ZIP _____

Number of Copies _____ @ $5.95 is $ _____
Enclosed is a check (or money order) in the amount of $5.95, payment in full, which includes postage costs. You may also charge to your VISA, Master Card or American Express card. Please include all necessary information.

Insert in envelope, **stamp** and **send** to:
LIFEPLAN
American Health and Nutrition
7 N. Pinckney, Suite 225
Madison, WI 53703

If you wish to receive a copy of LIFEPLAN FOR HEALTH AND FITNESS, fill out and mail this card.

Please send to the following address:

NAME _____

ADDRESS _____

CITY _____

STATE _____ ZIP _____

Number of Copies _____ @ $5.95 is $ _____
Enclosed is a check (or money order) in the amount of $5.95, payment in full, which includes postage costs. You may also charge to your VISA, Master Card or American Express card. Please include all necessary information.

Insert in envelope, **stamp** and **send** to:
LIFEPLAN
American Health and Nutrition
7 N. Pinckney, Suite 225
Madison, WI 53703

If you wish to receive a copy of LIFEPLAN FOR HEALTH AND FITNESS, fill out and mail this card.

Please send to the following address:

NAME _____

ADDRESS _____

CITY _____

STATE _____ ZIP _____

Number of Copies _____ @ $5.95 is $ _____
Enclosed is a check (or money order) in the amount of $5.95, payment in full, which includes postage costs. You may also charge to your VISA, Master Card or American Express card. Please include all necessary information.

Insert in envelope, **stamp** and **send** to:
LIFEPLAN
American Health and Nutrition
7 N. Pinckney, Suite 225
Madison, WI 53703

If you wish to receive a copy of LIFEPLAN FOR HEALTH AND FITNESS, fill out and mail this card.

Please send to the following address:

NAME _____

ADDRESS _____

CITY _____

STATE _____ ZIP _____

Number of Copies _____ @ $5.95 is $ _____
Enclosed is a check (or money order) in the amount of $5.95, payment in full, which includes postage costs. You may also charge to your VISA, Master Card or American Express card. Please include all necessary information.

Insert in envelope, **stamp** and **send** to:
LIFEPLAN
American Health and Nutrition
7 N. Pinckney, Suite 225
Madison, WI 53703

Important Notice

The information in this book is provided for educational purposes only and is meant to complement the advice and guidance of your doctor, not to replace it. Therefore the information herein is not meant to be used in diagnosis or treatment of any illness or disease.

**Please See Other Side
For Order Forms For Additional Books.**